Fifty Years of Healing:

Dr. Plechner's perspective on a half century of curing animals many had given up on

By
Dr. Alfred J. Plechner,
Doctor of Veterinary Medicine

Edited by
Kirk E. Nims
With the assistance of
Linda Blundell

Forewords by
Dr. Albert Simpson, DVM
Dr. Kathryn E. Calabria, DO

Fifty Years of Healing:
Dr. Plechner's perspective on a half century of curing animals many had given up on

Copyright © 2012 Dr. Alfred J. Plechner, D.V.M.

Printed by CreateSpace, Charleston, South Carolina, USA
[an Amazon.com company]

ISBN-10: 1453889590
EAN-13: 978-1453889596
Library of Congress Control Number: 2010915895
Createspace, North Charleston, SC

Printed in the United States
Made in the USA

This book is intended for information only. Please contact your own health care professional for specific recommendations and treatment. Health care providers interested in further information about the clinical studies and medical information contained herein should contact Dr. Plechner.

Contents

Contents

.

Editor's Foreword by Kirk E. Nims

I am a dog lover. Pure and simple, there is no way around it. I was born within days of my "nanny," Ellen, having delivered a litter of pups. Ellen was my grandmother's Irish setter. I was put with Ellen and her pups, and she took excellent care of me. I apparently took a particular liking to one of my pup brothers, and he was kept. Duke and I grew up together, and I am told that Duke was very patient with me as I used him to pull myself up to learn to walk and rode on his strong back as an infant. I tell people that I spoke Dog before Human, and find that I often prefer the company of dogs over socializing with most people.

For my seventh birthday, I was permitted to pick my own Airedale pup to raise and live with. I don't really remember why, at age six, I had decided that what I wanted most in the world was to have an Airedale puppy to raise, but it had to be an Airedale. He was Andy, bought from a local backyard breeder as a pet dog. Nobody fancy, just a good solid pure Airedale pup of a large size. As it turned out, he was Andy I, the first of my four Andys to date.

In July of 1996, at just short of his thirteenth birthday, Andy III passed away from the effects of congestive heart failure. He had lived a long, but sickly, life. He had a heart murmur and had a very touchy bowel. Some would say he had irritable bowel disease. He lived on a special feed and had a very bland diet. I kept him going and healthy by completely eliminating all stress from his life. When he got stressed, he would have "an episode" of gas and explosive, bloody diarrhea. Andy III was a very sweet and highly intelligent dog. Unlike his previous namesakes, Andy III did not have "hot spots" or other skin allergies. He was just cursed with this terrible bowel that completely controlled his life. I now know, in retrospect, that Andy III was a Plechner's Syndrome dog.

Andy III died just as we were commencing construction on our house in the woods south of Houghton Lake, Michigan. It was unfair to even consider getting another pup as we spent every waking moment either at work or getting ready to go "Up North" to build. So we waited.

As the construction ended, we began to discuss getting another Airedale. I looked into a rescue and came across Airedale Terrier Rescue and Adoption (ATRA). I completed an application and still looked into where I might find a good quality pet pup. As it turned out, the night that I went ahead and committed to a pup from a breeder, I got a phone call from Annette Hall of ATRA. She was in trouble and wanted to know if we could take a large Airedale named Miles as a short-term foster because her house was full up and Miles wanted NOTHING to do with the man of the house where she thought she would place him. Simply put, Miles would rather have eaten this man than live with him. Annette had checked us out already due to our application and, much to her surprise, Miles took an immediate liking to both Mike and me. Within minutes, it was clear that Miles thought that Mike was the best, and Mike would be his human.

On the evening of March 16, 1999, Sir Miles Doo Bop, the soon-to-be six-year-old, hundred-pound, almost thirty-inch-tall orphan from Cleveland, Ohio, came into our lives. There were many adventures with Sir Miles over his twelve years, and he went on to become, literally, world famous. People came to Michigan from Australia to meet him and visit.

Sir Miles also brought Dr. Alfred J. Plechner into our lives. On February 1, 2001, Miles bit Mike. For this, Miles went to jail and was on death row. During his quarantine period, Debbie Carley from Massachusetts found information about a veterinarian in California who was working wonders with dogs and had considerable success in helping dogs that for previously unexplained reasons had exhibited aggression. You see, Miles was a lover boy. He adored Mike. But at times, Miles would lose control of his demeanor and he would get ugly. At these times, we could see that he was not himself. His eyes would change, and it took a great deal to bring him back to being himself again; he would also shake his head and flap his ears.

I contacted Dr. Plechner, and as we talked, he assured me that he knew what was going on, so we arranged to have Miles' blood tested via an Endocrine/Immune 1 (EI1) panel at National Veterinary Diagnostic Services, a laboratory in Los Angeles. Miles was a Plechner's Syndrome dog. We put him on the oral hormonal balancing protocols, and within days we were beginning to see a different Miles. At the end of his life, Miles was walking around our neighborhood off lead, at Mike's side, with small children loving on him and hugging him. We had fixed him. He had been sick, and Dr. Plechner knew what was wrong and how to fix him.

Many Airedales have been helped due to our experience with Miles and Dr. Plechner. There is a Yahoo! Group devoted to Airedale (and other breed) owners who want to discuss and share information about the diagnosis and treatment of Plechner's Syndrome in our dogs. Right now, two of our Airedales are being treated for Plechner's Syndrome, and a third is hypothyroid. I have every confidence that Sir Miles II (he came back to us, but that is another whole story for another book) will come to develop into another Plechner's Syndrome Airedale. He is starting to get a bit grouchy again as he ages in this life.

In May 2001, Aemon Forrester, who lived with his Airedale pack and Sue and Bill at Wombat Bend in the Yarra Valley north of Melbourne, Australia, was stricken by a severe attack of autoimmune hemolytic anemia (AIHA). He was self destructing blood cells far faster than he could possibly produce them and was in critical condition in the local veterinary hospital. He had already been transfused three times when I called Dr. Plechner and asked him if he could suggest any treatment or care for Aemon, as the World Airedale Groups feared for his life. "Of course," was the response from Dr. Plechner. "Have Sue call me immediately with the information and put me in contact with Aemon's doctor." I called Sue and Bill and awoke them in the middle of the night with minimal apology. This was a matter of life or death, and they needed to start Aemon's treatment immediately if there was any chance of saving him. Sue immediately called Dr. Plechner and put him in contact with Aemon's doctor. In talking with Dr. Plechner over the next few days, as Aemon teetered on the brink of death, he kept telling me that he hoped that he had gotten to Aemon soon enough to push him off the fence he was sitting on to the **good** side. He had no serum test numbers as there were no laboratories in Australia that were capable of doing the endocrine and immune globulin studies that he usually has at hand during treatment. Dr. Plechner worked with his extensive experience, the available blood tests, packed cell volume studies, and Aemon's vitals as they slowly pushed him off dead center toward his return to good health. Aemon, much to everyone's joy, returned to good health and never had another AIHA attack.

We have helped with the cure of two German Shepherd dogs that I knew were sick with Plechner's Syndrome just based upon their reported symptoms. One of them lives with the president of Starting Over Airedale Rescue (SOAR). The other lives with our frequent dinner companions at a local restaurant. Dr. Plechner helped to save the life of our friend's Yellow Lab, Tad, who spent days in the hospital and was transfused due to an autoimmune hemolytic anemia attack. When I found out, I had his owner immediately contact Dr. Plechner for treatment. Tad turned around immediately after our veterinarians got the results of his EI1 panel back and Dr. Plechner advised them as to how they should proceed with his treatment. Tad's family said he was turning around in hours and got better day by day, and now, well over a year past his AIHA attack, he remains healthy and happy.

I have had an ongoing relationship with Dr. Plechner for over ten years now. We correspond and talk regularly. I count him as a friend. I know him to be kind, highly intelligent, and dedicated to his patients above and beyond all else. He is inquisitive and a very competent diagnostician. I consider him to be a medical genius. He has, through his intelligence, inquisitiveness, breadth of medical knowledge, vast clinical experience, and perseverance in finding cures for his patients, "discovered" not only what I have come to call Plechner's Syndrome, but also what I know to be a highly effective and safe treatment protocol that rebalances the endocrine system of affected animals.

What is Plechner's Syndrome? I wrote this definition and Dr. Plechner told me, upon reading it, that it was the concise description that on his own he had been trying to come up with for years.

> **Plechner's Syndrome** is an accumulation of a widely varying group of clinical signs and symptoms that characterize any of a variety of disease abnormalities or conditions that create a specific identifiable pattern in specific hormone and antibody levels in blood serum of several species of mammals. This syndrome is due to a damaged middle

layer adrenal cortex because of a genetic predisposition, environmental toxins, or aging. This damaged middle layer adrenal cortex in turn causes a reduction in active (working) cortisol, resulting in an elevated amount of estrogen to be produced by the inner layer adrenal cortex. Normal amounts of cortisol may be present; however, this cortisol can be defective or bound, and the same estrogenic effect may occur. The cortisol and estrogen imbalance usually presents itself as an altered immunity status with antibody depression present. This not only may result in malabsorption from the intestines, but also allows the immune cells to lose recognition of the body's own tissue and thus attack their own host. These changes in glandular performance allow for a variety of medical effects to occur, from allergies to irritable bowel disease, autoimmunity, uncontrolled tissue growth, and cancer.

The rest of this book will explain all of this in very great detail. Dr. Plechner has been treating animals with this disorder for many, many years. He has been doing so very successfully. The diagnostic blood tests work. The balancing protocols for the hormones work to safely and effectively return the serum level of the key hormones to mid-range level or as close to mid-range as can be achieved.

I am editing this book because I know this all works. I find that it is virtually a medical miracle that very sick animals can be returned to health with a blood test and the administration of some hormones in dosages designed to restore the daily blood levels of these essential hormones to normal levels.

Other veterinarians are beginning to awaken to the fact that there are serious medical issues around excessive estrogen being present in the bloodstreams of animals.

Steroid Profiles in the Diagnosis of Canine Adrenal Disorders Jack W. Oliver, Proceedings, 25th ACVIM Forum, pp. 471-473, Seattle, WA. 2007.

Hyperestrinism in Dogs

Hyperestrinism in dogs may be a new and emerging disease entity. In sample submissions to the Clinical Endocrinology Service (2005) at The University of Tennessee, 40% of adrenal panels had elevated estradiol levels present (>70 pg/ml).[29] In hyperestrinism cases, estradiol is the estrogen that is increased, ACTH stim and LDDS tests are usually normal for cortisol, thyroid function is normal or controlled, liver problems are frequent and typical (very elevated alkaline phosphatase, hepatomegaly, steroid hepatopathy, hyperechoic liver by ultrasound), PU/PD is frequent, panting may be present, hair/coat problems often are present, skin biopsy results suggest an endocrinopathy, there is no change in estradiol level in response to ACTH stim or LDDS tests as currently conducted, resistance to mitotane may occur and increase often occurs in response to trilostane. Effective treatment options for hyperestrinism in dogs is limited at the present time, and drugs that could be expected to be efficacious (aromatase inhibitors – excluding melatonin) often are limiting due to cost. Melatonin and phytoestrogen treatment may be effective for the above listed reasons. Mitotane will likely be effective if the source of estradiol is the adrenal tissues. Trilostane treatment frequently results in increased estradiol levels,[29] and this may be a reason why less than effective treatment with the drug sometimes occurs. +

The issue is that they have not awakened to the fact that it is the total of free estrogens in the bloodstream that causes the serious medical effects that are found in patients suffering from Plechner's Syndrome. The veterinary medical community needs to realize that there are safe and effective ways to rebalance the critical hormones to normal levels via the administration protocols that Dr. Plechner has developed over his years of clinical practice.

Dr. Plechner is a clinician. He works to heal sick patients day in and day out. He and a plethora of his patients and pet owners worldwide know that his diagnostic tests and treatment protocols work to restore health.

In June of 2001, I had the pleasure of discussing Dr. Plechner's work with Professor Clive Loveday, MD, who was at that time one of the faculty of the medical school at the University College of London. He is one of the foremost retrovirologists in the world and specializes in the study of HIV/AIDS. At that time, he told me that he believed that Dr. Plechner had discovered, through his clinical work, the critical measures of hormones in the blood system that were required to diagnose the imbalance that was apparently causing sickness. He further told me that he believed that Dr. Plechner had developed a safe set of protocols to administer replacement hormones to reestablish normal serum blood levels of the necessary hormones. In short, he believed, "This works." His challenge, as a medical scientist, was to go back to the laboratory and prove why it all works. He had to develop an understanding of the exact mechanism due to the imbalance that causes the illnesses and throws the immune system into disorder.

Eight years later, this remains the challenge to the scientific community. Those of us who have animals that are sick and getting sicker don't care about how or why this works. We are more than satisfied that our sick animals get well and stay well for extended lifetimes. We ask the medical scientists to please do the work to discover how all this works and, along the way, not to forget to give Dr. Alfred J. Plechner his due credit for having worked through these clinical miracles.

It would be good to take note of what Dr. P. M. F. Bishop, DM, states in his paper, delivered to the South London Medical Society. The paper is entitled "The History of the Discovery of Addison's Disease," published in the Proceedings of the Royal Society of Medicine, Vol. XLIII No. 1, 1950, Page 35, Sectional Page 1, Section of Endocrinology, October 26, 1949.

http://www.pubmedcentral.nih.gov/articlerender.fcgi?artid=2081266

> [Thomas] Addison, a morose and parochial physician diffidently describing first pernicious anaemia, and then, goaded on to more spectacular publication, produced a monograph which is still a masterpiece of clinical virtuosity, accurate and even now up to date in

every detail. This monograph, now one of the most famous in medical literature, was the subject of bitter controversy when it first appeared.

Cushing's syndrome was described by Harvey Cushing in 1932 in the *Bulletin of the Johns Hopkins Hospital*. He recorded 12 cases of this syndrome, and as he told me himself he travelled sometimes many hundreds of miles at short notice to be present at the post-mortem of some of the cases reported. Once again the eponym was applied by someone in another country (Bishop and Close), this time in England, and in this case it is possible that the eponym is well applied, for we still are not certain where the lesion lies, whether in the basophil cells of the pituitary, in the adrenal cortex, or whether, in some cases, there is a lesion at all. Cushing, at the time of his description of this syndrome, was the most famous neurosurgeon in the world. Whatever he might describe would instantly attract attention.

Cushing's discovery is not so very long ago. We are apt to think that Medicine has become so complicated, and so dependent on the laboratory and on team work, that no one individual can stand out as a giant among his peers in this rapidly progressing subject of endocrinology. This is surely not true.

Proceedings of the Royal Society of Medicine, Vol. XLIII, Page 42

Both of these famous clinical physicians described the disorders carrying their names based upon relatively few cases when compared to the many thousands of patients that Dr. Plechner has himself diagnosed and treated. Dr. Harvey Cushing used just twelve cases to describe his syndrome, and Dr. Thomas Addison used very few more in his papers and monograph describing Morbus Addisonii. I highly recommend reading the above paper in full and giving due consideration to a like paper, "The History of Cushing's Disease: A Controversial Tale," Dr. V. C. Medvei, MD, Journal of the Royal Society of Medicine, Volume 84, No. 6, Page 363, June, 1991. http://www.pubmedcentral.nih.gov/articlerender. fcgi?artid=1293286

When I encounter pet owners who are seeking diagnosis and treatment of their pets that are symptomatic for possible Plechner's Syndrome, I think of *Helicobacter pylori*. *Helicobacter pylori* are the bacteria that cause the majority of peptic ulcers. The article at http://www.search.com/reference/Helicobacter_pylori is highly informative. These bacteria were first discovered in 1875 in Germany.

> The bacterium was rediscovered in 1979 by Australian pathologist Robin Warren, who did further research on it with Barry Marshall beginning in 1981; they isolated the organisms from mucosal specimens from human stomachs and were the first to successfully culture them.

> The medical community was slow to recognize the role of this bacterium in stomach ulcers and gastritis, believing that no microorganism could survive for long in the acidic environment of the stomach.

> Before the appreciation of the bacterium's role, stomach ulcers were typically treated with medicines that neutralize gastric acid or decrease its production. While this worked well, the ulcers very often reappeared. A very often used medication against gastritis and peptic ulcers was bismuth subsalicylate. It was often effective, but fell out of use, since its mechanism of action was a mystery. Nowadays it is quite clear that it is due to the bismuth salt acting as an antibiotic. Today, many stomach ulcers are treated with antibiotics effective against *H. pylori*.

> In 1994, the National Institutes of Health (USA) published an opinion stating that most recurrent gastric ulcers were caused by *H. pylori*, and recommended that antibiotics be included in the treatment regimen.

> In 2005, Warren and Marshall were awarded the Nobel Prize in Medicine for their work on *H. pylori*.

> http://www.nlm.nih.gov/medlineplus/ency/article/000229.htm

I find this all particularly disturbing because all of the members of my great aunt's family suffered from peptic ulcers during the 1950s and onward. They even started a dairy goat farm because they got some comfort from drinking goat's milk along with their other treatments for their severe peptic ulcers. I first heard of the discovery of this cause of peptic ulcers in the late 1980s, and physicians were still prescribing antacids and performing surgery on their patients because they were certain that bacteria could not live in the stomach and these were the recognized, though completely wrong, treatment paradigms. It took an official opinion from the National Institutes of Health to get our doctors to stop their outdated modes of treatment.

When will the research on Plechner's Syndrome come before the National Institutes of Health or its counterpart in the world of veterinary medicine for an official opinion that will let the healing become more widespread and common? Please, let us get on with it.

It has been my personal pleasure to work on this project with Dr. Plechner and the other volunteer editors.

In the texts from Dr. Plechner which follow, I give you over to the only "slightly varnished and expurgated" Dr. Plechner. I have tried to let Dr. P's style and manner come through in these writings so that you can get a bit of the sense of the many conversations that I have had and many more that I look forward to in the future with this brilliant physician.

Foreword by Dr. Calabria

I would like to suggest that the title of this book be changed to *Our Pets, Ourselves*. When you understand how your pet gets sick, it helps you understand how you get sick. It is generally accepted that most illnesses can be traced back to a failing or malfunctioning immune system. Dr. Plechner's experimentation and research proves that the failure or malfunction can be traced back to the adrenal cortex, specifically the part that secretes cortisol.

The adrenal gland itself is misrepresented by its name, which implies it only makes adrenaline, which is well known for its role in the fight-or-flight reflex. Adrenaline is made in the center, or medulla, of the adrenal gland. However, the outer aspect, or cortex, of the adrenal gland makes steroid hormones like estrogen, testosterone, and DHEA, among others, as well as cortisol. Yes, cortisol is a steroid hormone. And in pill form it's known by several names: cortisone, hydrocortisone, methylprednisolone, (Cortef and Medrol are brand names), and by that most dreaded of all drug names, prednisone.

Prednisone has received a bad reputation by the accepted practice of prescribing it in very high doses, also known as pharmacologic doses. Such high doses can result in high blood levels. Over the long term, this can cause a lot of harm, and most people are aware of this. However, over the short term, this can be lifesaving, which is why it became an accepted practice.

William Jefferies, MD, wrote an excellent book called *The Safe Uses of Cortisol*, in which he discusses his years of experience in prescribing cortisone in physiologic doses. This is the drug dose that is needed when the adrenal cortex is not making enough cortisol to sustain health. Dr. Jefferies' book deals with human patients who had no or very poor adrenal function. He noted that one patient was given seventy milligrams of hydrocortisone four times daily for a week during a bout of pneumonia, and the patient's blood levels never went above normal.

In a normal functioning state, we (animals and people) often come into contact with viruses or bacteria that can cause pneumonia, skin infections, etc, but our immune system kicks in and we never know about it. Trouble occurs when the secretion continues for a prolonged period. This occurs during periods of prolonged stress.

We often think of emotional issues as a cause of stress and almost never consider pollution as stress. The causes of prolonged stress can, in fact, be due to pesticide or heavy metal exposure, or to poor quality nutrition, which can have xenoestrogens, food additives, coloring, preservatives, etc., which impair the function of individual cells. This impairment is a chronic, prolonged stressor when it is going on for weeks, months, and years.

Under these conditions of prolonged stress, when cortisol goes high, the thyroid gland will stop producing thyroid hormone. This is to prevent a condition known as thyrotoxicosis, which is to say, too much thyroid hormone. To prevent this condition, the system becomes hypothyroid, which is to say, too little thyroid hormone. In his book, *Hypothyroidism: The Unsuspected Illness*, Broda O. Barnes, MD, discussed each of the chronic diseases associated with aging as being caused by slightly low thyroid hormone levels over the course of many years.

Today, a lot of advertisements focus on blocking cortisol secretion because of an increased waistline. Under conditions of prolonged stress, during which cortisol levels are high and thyroid levels are low, people will have weight gain, usually in the midsection of the body. This abdominal "fat pad" is a result of years of chronic stress, where cortisol levels are elevated, often for more than ten years. After that amount of time the adrenal cortex is usually in a state of fatigue, and blocking it may be the wrong course of action. It depends on what the actual problem is and how the chosen treatment works inside the body.

Dr. Plechner's approach, however, puts a halt to the continued disease state, whether it is cancer, allergies, arthritis, autoimmune disorders, chronic infection, or chronic fatigue syndrome. It does not cure any of the endocrine-immune disorders, but it does control them and at the same time allow a return to healthy function.

In this book, you will find a guide to understanding how toxins and infections affect immune system functioning, how that malfunctioning leads to malnutrition, and subsequently, how illness results. Certainly there are many books on this subject. What's unique about this book is that it offers the reader information on how to figure out what's wrong. Once there is an understanding of the exact problem, steps can be taken to correct or control it. There is no other book like this anywhere, because no practitioner of any of the medical arts has ever totally figured out this aspect of the process. And this aspect is the crux of it all. It has certainly changed my practice of medicine for the betterment of my patients' health. To this I owe a debt of gratitude to Alfred J. Plechner, DVM.

Kathryn E. Calabria, DO
Long Island, New York

Foreword by Dr. Simpson

In today's veterinary medicine, changes in treatment, diagnosis, and pathophysiology usually come from research at our universities and schools of veterinary medicine.

This has not always been the case. In the late 1970s and early 1980s, pioneering work on adrenal and thyroid endocrinology and immune system links were postulated by Alfred Jay Plechner, DVM. Careful research and clinical observations uncovered the relationship between the endocrine system and the immune system, and how they manifested conditions that were thought before to be unrelated clinical diseases. In his first book, *Pet Allergies*, Dr. Plechner outlined the complicated interactions of cortisol, thyroid, total estrogen, and three main antibodies as they apply to allergies and intestinal disease. In Dr. Plechner's second book, *Pets at Risk*, he further linked endocrine-immune disorders to heredity and environmental toxins, as well as autoimmunity and cancer. Dr. Plechner dealt with these conditions every day as a practicing veterinarian. His research and findings were generated from his practice—not from a university—in the exam room, and they caused quite a lot of controversy and discussion.

Dr. Plechner has stood up to the task of defending his work and has seen it validated in many medical circles. In the last few years, he has been asked to lecture at several medical schools here in the U.S. and in England. Many health care professionals have adopted his procedures, achieving very positive results. He has a collection of published MD journals throughout the world. A compilation of these articles appears in his third book, entitled *Endocrine-Immune Mechanisms in Animals and Human Health Implications*. In addition to his clinical studies, he offers online seminars, two new unpublished books, and a medical dictionary for the pet owner.

As a practicing veterinarian, I personally have collaborated with Dr. Plechner on dozens of cases over the past fifteen years. These patients benefited from his work. Many of these cases had been given up on and were at the final chapter of their lives. Using his blood tests and carefully developed treatment protocols, many of these dogs and cats were returned to normal, healthy, happy lives.

Dr. Plechner's dedication to these pets is wonderfully evident. He is continuing to practice veterinary medicine, giving his gentle and caring touch and vast understanding of physiology for the benefit of those pets that are fortunate to be under his care.

Albert Simpson, DVM

Introduction

Large numbers of pets die or become sick before their time despite the best efforts of veterinarians. I believe that much of this has to do with hormonal imbalances that deregulate the immune system of animals, undermining their natural protection against illness and thus robbing them of good health and normal longevity.

Many "end-of-the-line animals" have been referred to me during my clinical practice. Their owners had been told that euthanasia was the only humane option left for their beloved pets. In some very advanced cases, those with permanent, irreversible damage having been caused, this has been true, but in a vast majority of situations there is hope for restoring these animals to good health because now there is a solution.

Many years ago as a young practitioner, I tried to figure out why so many patients were getting sick and not responding to standard treatments. My clinical work led me to a major hormone-based immune system disturbance that begins in the adrenal glands and goes on to create a ripple effect throughout the body's physiology. The conditions I was successfully treating were ranging from common allergies to reproductive failure to catastrophic autoimmune diseases and cancer. Through my clinical work over the years, identifying and correcting this endocrine system-based problem, I have developed a successful diagnostic and treatment protocol that has helped thousands of patients, not only in my own clinic, but also in many other veterinary clinics throughout the world.

The endocrine-immune imbalances I see are the result of an unsuspected deficiency, defect, or binding of cortisol. The pet-owning public, frequently, do not realize that they and their animals absolutely must produce a certain amount of natural cortisone to be able to live and function in a normal manner. Whether it is due to genetics, toxicity, stress, aging, or combinations thereof, many animals lack sufficient active cortisol. There is a general lack of medical knowledge regarding how to administer a cortisol replacement in order to safely regain the natural physiological level require for good health. "They don't teach us this in veterinary school," is often heard by owners with whom I consult when they talk with their own veterinarians, desperately seeking treatment for their seriously ill pets.

In animals and people needing long-term use of a cortisol replacement, it is advised that thyroid hormone must also be administered to guarantee that the cortisol is properly metabolized and does not accumulate in the system. I correct the cortisol deficiency by using very low doses (I would prefer using the term physiological as opposed to therapeutic dosages) of a cortisol replacement that is the pharmaceutical equivalent of the body's naturally occurring cortisol, along with thyroid hormone, depending on the species I am working with (personal communications and clinical experience supports not using the natural forms of cortisol.)

I believe that good medical practice is a blend between Eastern and Western medicine, including proper nutrition, supplementation, exercise, other stress reducers, and sleep. This, then, is what I like to call "Wholistic" medicine. Many medical practitioners, unfortunately, focus on the trees in front of them and miss the overall view of the forest.

The rebalancing hormone protocol has been extremely safe and effective when followed as directed on a long-term basis by pet owners. As a clinician, my patients are my primary concern. For this reason, I have not conducted controlled studies where one group of patients receives proper therapy and the other group receives a placebo. I will never deny proper treatment to a suffering patient.

Finally, if the identification and proper replacement protocol is carefully followed, this program can significantly and rapidly improve the health status of even very sick animals. It is also an approach that has significant insights for the treatment of human illnesses.

I have found that retirement was not all it is cracked up to be, and with overwhelming requests for me to make myself available, I have returned to practice and will be doing consulting for the general public and health care professionals. I also welcome communication from health care professionals who are interested in exploring the role of endocrine-immune imbalances in the good health of their patients.

I can be contacted for consultations at my website, http://drplechner.com .

Biography

I was born on April 4th, 1938, at an area called Three Tree Point on Puget Sound in the state of Washington. I can actually remember when I was four years old and received my first football. Since I had no other children as playmates, I used Puget Sound as a playmate. I knew, as a child, the Sound had its tides coming in and going out. So I picked a good time to play ball with the Sound. I knew if I threw my football into the Sound, it would surely come back. As you might imagine, I spent many waking moments waiting for my football to come floating back. Obviously, my football never came back. This was my first introduction into the world of reality.

To amuse myself, as I aged a couple of years, my parents allowed me to use an old rowboat as long as I wore a life preserver and stayed within sight of the house. The baby whales were all over the Sound at different times. We referred to them as black fish. The baby whales played around my rowboat and actually let me pet them. I am lucky their mothers never got upset with me.

I worked very hard catching small frogs for the bass fishermen and got paid a nickel apiece for them. I had hoped to make enough money to buy a radio-controlled car. My dad read to me about the little Japanese babies that were involved in the war and had no diapers and had to use newspaper instead. My dad helped me mail my life savings to the Seattle Times to buy diapers for the babies. The Times editors were nice enough to do a picture and article on my donation.

I continued with my rowboat adventures, and each year a very large white whale would spend some time in the Sound. People called it Orca, but it really was not. I remember its size, and it was gigantic. It was three times larger than a beluga whale.

After a time, we moved into town because my dad had horrible allergies and severe asthma. He was somewhat bedridden. He had been a great fisherman, when he was feeling well enough to go. I loved to go to Matthews Creek, which was close to the house. The creek came directly out of Lake Washington. I would catch salmon and trout and bring them home to show my dad in hopes that he would be proud of me. Unfortunately, he would accuse my mom of buying the fish for me so that he could be proud of me. Another reality check.

The next reality check was about to happen. One afternoon I was playing in the alley behind my house when a car came speeding up the alley and proceeded to run over my four-year-old sister. I was seven years old at the time. The next-door neighbors were both physicians and were home at the time. They wrapped my little sister in a blanket and headed to the nearest hospital. The interns and residents were in a meeting and too busy to see her despite her massive head trauma. By the time we reached the next hospital, she had died. What a great example for a seven-year-old to realize that taking the Hippocratic Oath must mean that you are a **hypocrite**. Reality is really getting tough! My mom and dad adopted a little girl we named Cathy. Everything returned to normal, as well as normal could be.

One afternoon when I was eleven years old, my dad had gone to the hospital for an injection of a bronchiole dilator called aminophyline. As you might guess he had a terrible reaction and died within a few minutes. When I came home from school, I was told that my dad was dead. Guess I am batting zero at this point. I soon became the man of the family. I guess I was lucky to have any childhood at all. I did escape from reality by playing classical music on the piano. I eventually took a total of fourteen years of instruction and played many concerts, but like many other things, my music became so intensely personal that I really only wanted to play for myself, with no audience. I worked very hard to get through school and support myself. We eventually moved from Seattle to Los Angeles so my mom could begin real estate school. I worked for Ralph's Market evenings and all day Saturdays and Sundays. I spent my summers working in my uncle's wholesale grocery warehouse in Portland, Oregon. Weekends I spent in Seaside. At the age of twelve, I worked for the Seaside Clam Company catching red-finned surf perch and salmon. I was paid ten cents a pound for the perch and twenty-five cents a pound for salmon.

Mom got her real estate license, and I figured out another additional way for "the man of the family" to make money. I raised orchids, 365 different species, and sold them as corsages at UCLA and USC for special events.

I also worked for the Osaki family, training trees in small dishes, called bonsai. It was very relaxing to do, and when I created a special bonsai, I would show the Osaki grandparents. They would admire the small tree and then politely bow to me, which meant they liked the results. I also did wet and dry gardens for people and created some greatly admired Japanese gardens. I actually did this for my mom in her backyard. I built a large covered patio with the entire back of it as a skylight. On the entire east wall, I did the same. On that wall I had huge boards covered in redwood bark. To this bark, I attached outside orchids and many species of bromeliads. All were wrapped in sphagnum moss and attached to the bark walls. In the back of the patio were my other species of orchids. A transparent wall and door allowed people to view and enjoy the flowers without having to enter the greenhouse. I built a large koi pond for Mom and built a bridge out of lotus bud knobs that bridged the pond, giving access into the patio across the pond. I also built a huge waterfall that created further peacefulness. Many people came to see the garden and patio. One day, the *Los Angeles Times* called my mom and asked if they might take pictures. The entire garden and patio made two colored pages in the home and garden section of the Sunday edition of the *Los Angeles Times*.

While working, I attended Los Angeles High School, where I wrestled and played football. I became head of the Varsity Lettermen's Society as a junior and, in 1956 as a senior, I was elected as the Boys Division President of my high school. I had been sent to Boys State in California as a junior in 1955 to help me become a better Boys Division President. Believe me, it was a wonderful experience that I really appreciated.

After five years of hard work, I applied to medical school so that I could help stop unnecessary medical tragedies such as those that befell both my dad and little sister.

In 1961, I was accepted to attend medical school at a major, highly regarded, Midwestern school of medicine. My mom did not want "the man of the family" to leave, but it was my time. I enjoyed medical school for my first year and was looking forward to becoming a pediatrician. While at medical school, my greatest pleasure was to walk a mile down to a little Italian fruit stand. Once there, I would buy a big, juicy, red apple and eat it on the way home.

At the end of my first year in medical school, I developed a horrible upset gut. The Dean of Men attributed my medical problems to freshman nerves.

After losing forty pounds and a lot of my hair, I looked at myself in the mirror (after having been given a treatment of two weeks of paregoric), and said, "Self, you are going to die." I went to see the Dean of Men the next morning, and I was so dehydrated, I spoke with a click. He said to me, "You could go into public health! It would be much less stressful." I flew home the next day, and I will always remember my mother and grandmother hugging each other and quietly sobbing because I looked like I had just come from a concentration camp.

I went to see my physician, who, with serum titers and my clinical symptoms and with just good medical diagnostic skills, said, "You have typhoid fever." My physician was livid that this third-world disease could have been missed in a student at this high-powered medical school! But, as we all know, sometimes we are too close to the picture, and it often takes someone else to properly diagnose the problem. The dean said that I should come on back and speak with my professors to figure out how to catch up with my classmates. Most of my professors were Nobel Prize winners in their respective fields. So, each professor told me that he or she taught the best class in the country, and I should take the other professors' classes in summer school. I went back to the dean about what was said. He told me to rest up and then come back next year and join the February class, but, if I decided not to, he would have an open acceptance for me whenever I wanted to come back.

Now at home recuperating and feeling better, I took my English Bulldog, Moose, to see my veterinarian. When my vet saw me he said, "I bet you hated medical school." I told him that I really did not, but it was like getting a PhD in a basic science. I have always wanted to be a clinician. My vet disappeared for a few minutes and when he returned, he had a phone in his hand and said, "There is someone on the phone who would like to speak with you." It was the dean of the veterinary medical school at the University of California at Davis. He asked me if I would like come up to UC Davis to speak with him. The more I thought about it, the better it sounded. The next day, I drove to Davis, and it turned out that both he and I were doing similar research studies. He asked me if I would like to join his fall class. He said to think about it. I did, and two weeks later, I called and accepted his offer. I never even had to apply. I started veterinary school in the fall of 1962 and graduated in August of 1966.

Paula the Marmoset

While I went to UC Davis School of Veterinary Medicine, I lived in North Hall, which was a designated living quarters for veterinary students and those studying for their PhDs in related subjects.

At the time, I had a wonderful white-lipped marmoset I called Paula. She was a wonderful small creature that I loved dearly. When I came back from classes, Paula was always there to greet me. As I would study at night, she would watch me and sleep on my lap. She was my family and little friend in my dorm room.

Often she would wait and watch for me to come home at night. One day, she heard footsteps in the dorm hallway and began to whistle as she always did when I was about to open the door and enter the room.

Unfortunately, these footsteps were from the dorm maintenance man, Malcolm. When he heard Paula whistle, he was sure a student was razzing him. He entered my room, saw Paula, and immediately called the campus police, to let them know that there was an ape in North Hall.

I came home from my last class to find out what had happened. Thankfully no one tried to remove Paula from my room. After all, she was a dangerous ape of twelve ounces.

The next morning I was called into the Dean of Men's office to explain myself.

I stated that I was a veterinary student studying primates and primate behavior, which I thought was an important part of my training. At the time, nothing like this was offered in this school of veterinary medicine.

The Dean of Men told me that Paula could no longer live with me. The entire event was so wrong, but I could not buck the system at that time; not then, as I can and do now.

I was told that I had Christmas vacation to place Paula. I did so with some very supportive people, but in spite of their care, Paula missed me, as I missed her. Living with me was the only home that she really knew. I wanted to see her on spring break in order to see how my little companion was doing and let her know that soon she could come home. When I went to surprise her, I was told that she had died. She had never recovered from leaving me. You can imagine how I felt, hoping that once I had graduated from vet school, I could again provide the home that she knew and loved.

The people who were the temporary caretakers of Paula had never called me to let me know that she had given up on life. They meant well, but obviously it was not enough.

Yes, I went back to my classes in vet school, but with a little different perspective.

The maintenance man, Malcolm, continued his job, with no mention of what he had caused. He could have cared less. Weekly, he would pass out clean sheets and towels to all of us for our rooms. Yes, we paid money for his wonderful service. It was not free. Several of my friends were very upset about Paula and vowed they would get even with Malcolm. Apparently, he worked during the week and not on the weekend.

What occurred was really something. My friends placed a calf, with diarrhea, with food, in Malcolm's closet with all the linens and towels for the weekend. They checked routinely on the calf to make sure the calf was all right. Sunday night my friends removed the calf from Malcolm's linen room and returned the calf back to the campus meadow. You can imagine what Malcolm's closet and linens looked like Monday morning. I thanked my friends for the "don't get mad, get even," but my heart was still very heavy for the loss of Paula.

She is definitely one reason why I care so much and why I will do anything I can do to help all my animals even though I could not help Paula.

Paula was named after my grandmother Paula, who acted as my real mother.

I think the statement that comes to mind is that you can achieve anything you want to, but it might not be right for you. I have run into many brick walls, but now I hope that I am a little bit smarter. Reality has gotten better. The second Christmas vacation, as a sophomore at UC Davis, I came home for the holidays. My mother had a lump in her left breast that had been found by a mobile cancer unit. She was to be rechecked in one month. I immediately called our family physician and had Mom in for surgery the next day. At this time, she was fifty-two years old with no family history of any kind of cancer.

The surgeons removed my mother's left breast plus her axillary lymph node. Frozen sections of the mass, at the time of surgery, revealed the presence of a malignant mammary tumor. Next, the surgeons took out both adrenal glands and irradiated both ovaries to reduce the risk of an "estrogenic effect," which not only caused the original tumor but could also cause it to spread. While I watched closely, I remember, with replacing the two types of adrenal hormone—glucocorticoid and mineral corticoid—she did well for four years.

Soon thereafter, while I was working on the cortisol, thyroid, estrogen connection, my mother began to seriously decalcify. She would be in bed, cough or sneeze, and fracture the bones in her spine and ribs. It was a horrible thing to witness. As her plight continued, I was aware of a thyroid imbalance that often, if not always, accompanies a cortisol-estrogen imbalance. At this point of my searching, I realized that the thyroid was bound and, as the daily dose of steroids was given, due to this thyroid hormone blockage, everyday there remained a residue of cortisol. So after a number of days, the regulatory amounts of controlling cortisol went from a physiological dose level to a harmful, pharmacological overdose.

Medically, my mother, besides the pathological fractures she sustained, was cold all the time and began to lose her hair. Her axillary temperatures were subnormal, even though her thyroid hormones were normal in tests, and she continued to decalcify. I spoke to my mother's physician, who agreed that trying thyroid supplementation on my mom could not hurt. Mom felt better immediately upon taking the thyroid hormone. Her temperature started to rise, and the decalcification stopped. Eventually, she began to re-calcify. On the adrenal and thyroid replacements, she lived until she was eighty-eight years of age, and just "went to sleep" one day.

To this day, total estrogen testing is not being done in 99 percent of human and veterinary laboratories. The lack of transference of thyroid hormone due to imbalanced or deficient cortisol also is not usually recognized. Testing for high total estrogen is not only not being done, but the realization of the fact that high-serum estrogen binds both thyroid hormones [T3 and T4] is not being practiced routinely by health care specialists for either people or animals.

It will be up to you to ask for these tests to be done because doctors and veterinarians are not taught these endocrine facts in medical school. If a laboratory cannot do these tests for total estrogen, etc., then please ask your health care professional to find a lab that can. Realize you will be wasting your money otherwise, but, what is more important, you may be losing your life or the life of your pet.

The Battle of Stonewood Meadows

For many years, I have been seriously involved with wildlife management on a now-and-then basis.

Biography

Besides having a wildlife rehabilitation center that I ran, I was the volunteer research immunologist for the Bighorn Sheep Society for the State of California. I was doing my Plechner's Syndrome testing for the bighorn sheep in the early 1970s to try to determine which rams and ewes would create lambs in the future that would be healthier. I was able to take blood samples from the lambs and ewes we caught under our nets with apple butter bait. The rams we took from a helicopter, with tranquilizer darts.

I was able to review the results from the lab tests and decide if this would be a good genetic transplant for Independence, California. It definitely was. Charlie Jenner and I were the volunteer veterinarians on this particular project. The young man spearheading this effort was Jim DeForge.

Charlie, Jim, and I flew up to the University of California at Davis to help create a program for Jim to get his PhD in bighorn sheep research management.

While this was occurring, it became very apparent to me, and many other people involved in saving captured wildlife species in the Santa Monica Mountains, that most of the captured wildlife in Los Angeles County were being released in Los Padres National Forest or were being euthanized.

I decided that if I could find a piece of property in a significant ecological area of the Santa Monica Mountains, I could provide Los Angeles County, the state fish and game department, and the federal fish and game agency with a place to relocate indigenous species.

I was looking for a significant environmental area that was conducive for wildlife at the base of the Santa Monica Mountains on the valley side of the mountains that contained year-round water and good wildlife habitat.

I knew if I could find property like this, I could definitely enhance the plants to provide great forage for the relocated species to feed upon, and they could remain there until they felt safe enough to return to their own natural environment in the mountains.

I spoke to one of my clients, who was a realtor, and I asked her to look for a parcel for me. She said she had twenty-seven acres next to her that was for sale. The property was on either side of Cold Creek at the base of Cold Canyon, which covered about ten thousand acres.

This was a natural for me and was not expensive, so I proceeded. I wanted to create a self-sufficient wildlife preserve that did not need to rely on donations to survive.

Since I was at the time the Assistant Director of Wildlife for the Topanga Las Virgenes Resource Conservation District, I had a tremendous support group to help me with my project. They gave me the telephone number for the head of soil conservation in the United States Department of Agriculture. His name was Bobby Gaines. He designed a soil conservation plan for me such that I could not only treat and release indigenous wildlife species, but at the same time, Mr. Gaines would teach me to be a better steward of the soil.

I felt that if I did a farm-based wildlife preserve, the sales of fruits and nuts would support the project without counting on any donations. My young sons helped me plant two hundred apricot and almond trees. My boys also helped me plant ten thousand grape cuttings and helped put out irrigation for the soon-to-become grapevines.

I had no money and was fortunate enough to buy grape cuttings from the Sisquok Ranch just east of Santa Maria, California. The workers in the fields knew that I could not tell with the horizontal buds on the cuttings which way was up or down. So, the workers charged me a nickel for each cutting and cut the bottom of the cuttings flat, which meant that part went into the ground, and a point at the top of the cuttings that pointed to heaven.

I have always been guided in my adventures even though sometimes I questioned my direction.

I knew I had been led correctly because Jay, one of my sons, helped me dig the first hole for the first grape cutting, and there was a rock structure at the bottom of the hole. Once I was able to remove this "rock," it turned up a half of a Shumach Indian bowl. I knew we had been guided home.

Every Friday night I would drive my boys and myself up to my project. I had a king-sized mattress in the back of my truck for my boys and myself to sleep on with our sleeping bags, and we had a cooler with food and water.

They would sleep all night, and I would get up every hour to change the irrigation lines. In the early morning, it was really cold, so I would drive my boys down to Ventura Boulevard, where there was a diner. Bob, the owner, would make special animal pancakes for the boys plus eggs and bacon for all of us. The hot chocolate and coffee, plus the food, got us ready for another day at the preserve.

The boys and I will always remember lying in the back of my truck and watching a huge meteor scream across the sky that was so close to earth and us, it must have hit the earth somewhere.

Another time, we were awakened by a rattling of our food chest. It turned out to be some young raccoons we had released a few weeks ago. They must have decided that the frogs, crayfish, and various bugs did not taste as good as our peanut butter and jelly sandwiches.

The plants were doing well, and so were my sixteen beehives, so I decided to further help support my independent wildlife preserve. I was able to sell a five-gallon container of honey for fifty bucks. But unfortunately for my bees, there was not enough food for them to eat during the winter; I decided to grow from seed two hundred lemon eucalyptus trees to provide food for the bees during November, December, and January.

Since the trees were very young and could not produce enough blooms to help sustain my bee population yet, I decided to move my beehives home with me. There were lots of blooms in the mid-Wilshire district of Los Angeles.

My bees were doing just great, and I thought I had found a great way to feed my honeybees and sell honey during the winter to help support my self-sufficient wildlife preserve.

WRONG!

You could see this huge funnel of bees coming back into my yard with their pollen from the neighborhood. You need to know that I had my sixteen beehives in the backyard of my small house, located on Orange Drive. For those of you who do not know this area, it is right in the middle of Los Angeles between 6th Street and Wilshire Boulevard.

Unfortunately for me and my bees, they would lay bee pollen on the executives' fancy cars at the Carnation building, close to my house, and someone apparently decided that the bees were the problem.

The next day, the county bee inspector began driving up and down the street looking for possible beehives. Unfortunately for me and my wildlife project, he saw my bees funneling down into my backyard. As it turned out, I did not want my bees to die, so I thought it best to give my bees and their hives to the inspector to keep and have them flourish.

During that time, I had been picking up wild beehives from UCLA, and one day, I was in a hurry to get the hive and I received thirty bee stings. I had my older son, Jay, with me, plus the head of the entomology unit. As I pulled up in front of the entomology building on campus, I took my truck out of gear, pulled the parking brake on, and passed out. Needless to say, I scared both of them to death. Soon after, I decided to find another way to make money for my wildlife project.

Soon thereafter, having been working seven days and two nights a week for as long as I could remember, I received an invitation to go to Colorado for ten days and actually exist at ten thousand feet, looking at elk, deer, bear, and all kinds of other wildlife species. I definitely was ready and could not resist the opportunity.

Biography

The air was so thin at that elevation, if we decided to start a fire for a barbeque, we had to use a hair dryer. Because of the high altitude, our pancakes turned into muffins. Pretty neat! After having had this wonderful experience, I will never forget what happened next.

I returned home on October 8, 1978, and had a telegram waiting for me from Evel Younger, Attorney General of the State of California, stating that if I continued working on the wildlife preserve, I would be fined ten thousand dollars per day and put in jail.

"What the hell is this about?"

I was told that I was in violation of the California Coastal Act.

I have a greenbelt wildlife project that complements the Coastal Act. Why would they take me on? All I ever wanted to do was to set up a farm-based wildlife preserve for the agencies and private citizens to relocate indigenous species in the Santa Monica mountains.

I had been licensed not only by the Fish and Wildlife Service federally but was also licensed by the California Department of Fish and Game and was implementing a USDA soil conservation plan. On my twenty-seven acres, I only wanted to build one residential home and a treatment barn where I could rehabilitate and release indigenous wildlife species.

You know, I thought I still lived in America, but maybe not!

I contacted the State Coastal Commission to find out what was going on. I was given a staff person, who was telling everyone what a bad person I am. Her name was Janice Ann Potter. When I contacted her on the phone she said, "We got ya." I asked her, "What does that mean?"

She said that I did not meet the requirements for the AVCO subdivision laws. I asked what does that mean? She said you do not have enough lumber on the ground to meet the requirements of our California Coastal Commission.

What lumber?

I asked her what the commission wanted of me. She said, "We want an easement, the full length of the creek bottom."

I asked myself, "Why is this happening?"

I was trying to do something good for the wildlife and the wildlife agencies, at my own expense. I am a licensed veterinarian and a definite part of the greenbelt in the California Coastal Act. I had no idea why this was happening.

The local homeowners' association, plus all the horse people organizations, the Sierra Club, and the Nature Conservancy were all against my project.

I own my own property. Apparently, I have no constitutional rights here in California and, as this bureaucratic nightmare plays out, you will see I was never in the coastal zone in the first place and they had no jurisdiction. Needless to say, they and the attorney general continued the persecution of me, my family, and my wildlife preserve.

A so-called neighbor who lived down the road borrowed his brother-in-law's loader and took his child for a ride down a steep embankment with the bucket of the loader high in the air. Unfortunately, the loader toppled face first, pinning the neighbor under the loader. When I was contacted regarding the emergency, I loaded up my TD 18 down on a large trailer. I took my bulldozer to the accident site, and I was able to free the neighbor. This neighbor apparently was part of the group of people who were trying to stop my project.

I could not live on my land and treat damaged wildlife species there because I could not get a coastal permit unless I gave an easement to the California Coastal Commission the length of the stream bottom. This entire area is a significant ecological area. Why then, would these so-called environmentalists want horse and hiking trails through a year-round stream?

Can you imagine the wildlife, deer, cougar, raccoons, and possums, besides the nesting ducks, quail, and a myriad of other indigenous species, having their protected habitat invaded by a bunch of amateur human beings while the wildlife needs to wait and hopefully be allowed to get a drink out of the creek, which hopefully is not full of horse feces and human urine?

During the week, since I was not allowed to live on my own property, people would trespass. They tore down my grape stakes, put cornmeal into the diesel tank of my bulldozer, and did whatever else they could do to destroy my hope of developing a wildlife preserve on my own property!

The wife of the fireman I rescued from under the loader called my neighbor to let her know that their group was going to rent a huge bulldozer [D9] and were intending to entirely destroy my wildlife project. She said, "I do not like Dr. Plechner, but I think this is wrong." It was interesting that her husband was head of the fireman's union at the time, and I had so many firemen friends who were totally supportive of what I was doing. Why was this?

Once my supportive neighbors got wind of this large bulldozer and what these people intended to do, all my neighbors called all the heavy equipment rental places to let them know that if they dropped off a piece of equipment at Monte Nido and Old Mulholland Highway in Calabasas, there was a good chance I would bury the driver and the piece of equipment.

I took some time off to prepare for the battle. I had my big bulldozer placed in a position where I was going bury the operator and the piece of equipment. I had had enough, and it was now time to go for the throat!

Fortunately, or unfortunately, a nice neighbor who lived up the road, Tiffy Cappel, was dating one of the LA County supervisors, Baxter Ward. Supervisor Ward called the Malibu sheriff, who came out to my property and said, "You really do not want to do this because even if he trespasses, if you damage him or his equipment, you will have to pay for it."

Fortunately, I had done a lot of work with a county animal care officer, Marty Broad. We had this great wildlife coalition going. If feral dogs ran a deer into the ocean in Malibu, the lifeguards would try to haze the deer into the beach with their surfboards. If this did not work, then the sheriff would take out the helicopter and do the same thing.

Officer Broad would be on the beach to restrain the animal and bring it to me for a quick exam and possible injection for infection and stress, and then he released them on my wildlife preserve. Marty asked me what he might do to help my situation. I indicated to Marty what was occurring with neighborhood trespassing and vandalism.

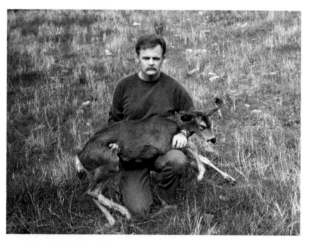

Dr. Alfred Plechner during the time of the Battle of Stonewood Meadows with injured black-tailed deer.

What then occurred was that whenever the sheriff flew out, if possible, they would fly up Cold Canyon over my property, and if they saw anyone on my preserve, they would bullhorn them out to Mulholland Highway, where the California highway patrol would take over.

The new police activity and arrests definitely made people think twice before they decided to trespass and vandalize my preserve.

Thank heaven for people like Marty and all those other law enforcement agencies that went out of their way to help wildlife, not because they have to but because they care.

Getting back to the "environmental recreationists," the homeowners, environmentalists, and equestrian groups had only begun demonstrating their lack of concern for the environment and probably the most fragile segment of our earth, the wildlife.

They again trespassed and took pictures of a huge split rock on the top of my preserve and took pictures somewhere of a dirt trench; they went in front of the State Coastal Commission and represented these photos as evidence as to where I fed my wildlife. Forget all the native forage I planted for these various species.

This group, including the Monte Nido Homeowners' Association, accomplished their purpose.

The California Coastal Commission decided that I was such a bad person that they would never allow me to testify in front of them, ever. Fortunately, I had a client who was one of the two people in the Department of Justice who uncovered the Watergate scandal. At this same time, Roger Osenbaugh and his partner were on President Reagan's environmental committee and, while attending the particular state coastal hearing, they heard the verbiage that was used against me at the California Coastal Commission meeting. The next day they called me to get some answers.

When they understood what was going on, they volunteered to help me. It is important to say that all the people involved never took a penny for their involvement. They believed in the project.

Richard Kirshner was the client involved with uncovering the Watergate scandal, and with his wonderful gravelly voice, he persuaded the California Coastal Commission to let me testify in front of them.

You can imagine my feelings as to testifying in front of the commission that I believed in, but there I was, not knowing why they were trying to stop a project that was supposed to be part of the Coastal Act.

Fifty Years of Healing

I forced myself to leave my veterinary practice, leaving patients that needed help, to drive to San Francisco to appear in front of these political idiots with their agenda to hurt the environment. Why was this happening? It was like having a nightmare while you are still awake.

I drove up to San Francisco to the state commission inquisition, and Roger was there to help me. I was totally out of my element as a poor veterinarian only trying to do something decent for wildlife and the coastal zone on my own property. Why the hell were these people against what I was doing?

When I got to the commission hearing, I was told that I had already lost without the commission even hearing me. A staff person brought me notes from five different coastal commissioners who believed in me. Their notes were telling me how to sue the commission on various different points.

I needed to get back to my practice and my patients that needed my help.

I did not know what to do. My wife called me a fool and said I should give them the easement. Eventually a divorce occurred based upon another problem, and I was granted custody of both my boys in 1978.

By this time, I was so frustrated with the neighbors and the commission that my boys and I built a flagpole in the middle of the wildlife preserve. We used native rock and had a brass plate made for the base of our new flagpole, and we dedicated it to the loss of our constitutional rights, in the state of California, in the coastal zone. My boys, six and nine years of age, proudly raised our country's flag; our flagpole violated not only three coastal codes but four county codes as well.

We notified the media about why we were doing this, and it turned out to be a total media blitz.

The next day, on the front page of the *Los Angeles Times*, was an article by the Coastal Commission and their staff person stating that the Smith Act had just been passed, which allows a person to build a flagpole without a coastal permit. As far as Dr. Plechner was concerned, "We don't like him, and we wish he would go away." Trust me, my boys and I will never "go away" from an injustice like this.

Soon thereafter, the Nature Conservancy contacted me to see what they could do to stop me from doing another media blitz. They definitely did not want any future problems for environmentalists.

At this same time, our lieutenant governor, Leo McCarthy, was on board. The legislature in Sacramento knew there was a veterinarian in southern California that was, in their words, "Kicking the ass of the Coastal Commission."

Don't you kind of wonder why all of this occurred? I sure did.

I finally realized what was happening. All the environmentalists, horse and hiking groups, Nature Conservancy, Sierra Club, along with the California Coastal Commission, were misusing their powers to set up the future Santa Monica National Park.

My preserve reminded them of the trail that they built on the top of Cold Canyon so that these wonderful recreational environmentalists could hike and ride their horses and look down upon what used to be a golden eagle nesting spot. The eagles left their nest, for good, for good reason.

I also reminded the true conservation groups that when hay is purchased from the high desert of Arizona and Nevada, and when you feed this to a horse, if you allow that horse to go through a bog or wet area like a creek or stream, the noxious weed seeds will not be digested in the hay and will be passed out in the feces. In twenty years, our native riparian areas will represent the plants that grow in the high desert environment of Arizona and Nevada.

The California Coastal Commission and all the environmental groups were trying to stop all development of any sort in the Santa Monica Mountains so the state or federal government could own it all. Their obvious feeling was, as part of their larceny, "The hell with the wildlife."

Environmental recreation seems to be the most important thing to this uneducated commission and the other associated groups. Their overall plan was to not only steal as much land from innocent people in order to create the Santa Monica National Park, but to also hook up all the significant ecological areas for hiking and horseback from Griffith Park to Malibu. By the way, they call this the Backbone Trail. In doing so, their trail maps would represent the backbones of all the wildlife that died as a result of their trails.

Soon thereafter, I received an article that said I was a builder and a builder developer. I was told it came from the new prospective superintendent for the Santa Monica National Park. This letter went to President Reagan and, as I understand it, President Reagan sent him back to Colorado.

A trail was eventually worked out to route the horse people, hikers, and environmentalists on a dirt road outside of my wildlife preserve and out of the creek.

I have been told that the Battle of Stonewood Meadows verses the California Coastal Commission set precedents for wildlife over recreation in the State of California in the coastal zone.

It is important to remember that good land use is important for hikers, horse riders, dirt bikes, and off-road vehicles, and there is room for all, but you do need to respect those small ecological pockets that our fragile wildlife still call home.

It was really difficult fighting these people while at the same time trying not to create a paper trail for the builders to follow on my shirttails and ruin the coastal zone, which I am not only part of but also do believe in.

"What Ever Happened to Stonewood Meadows?"

As it turned out, my grapes were elegant. A young man who had worked for me for a couple of years wanted to become a veterinarian. But his talents were already preconceived. He went to UC Davis to become a great winemaker—an enologist. He had gold medals in winemaking as a sophomore. Upon graduation, he went to work for Bogle Vineyards. He really did put them on their feet financially with wonderful wines that were drinkable soon and not in ten to twenty years.

I was the vintner that grew our vines, and my sons and I would decide when to harvest. Then I would rent a refrigeration truck, pick all the grapes with my sons, and fill up the truck with barrels filled with Cabernet, Zinfandel, and Johannesburg Riesling. After the twenty-eight-foot truck was filled on the bed, I would stack plywood over the barrels and do another stack.

I would then drive the grapes up to Clarksberg, to Bogle Vineyards. Mark would make the wine, and he and I would split the cases of production. I then drove home my bottles of Calabasas Cellars and sold the wine to different wine merchandisers. This was how I was going to support my bird-of-prey center on the wildlife preserve. The *Los Angeles Times* loved the wine and included me in their wine and food section in their Sunday edition for quite awhile. Liquor Barn had ordered some wine for a store out in the San Fernando Valley, and my poor son, Jay, went to deliver our wines. When he got there, he was told, "Get the hell out of my store! I do not want any more of your cr**py wine here!" All my son was doing was what the Liquor Barn had told us to do in order to help us to fund our self sufficient wildlife relocation center.

The label was the head and neck of an American eagle and called Calabasas Cellars.

The Los Angeles times revered our cabernet at that time.

Soon thereafter, the Liquor Barn and Irvine Ranch Markets bought all my wine, which would have given me money to build my bird-of-prey center, and then they went bankrupt. What do you do now?

While I was also trying to make a difference for pets, I was deciding, in practice, how I could identify whether a dog or cat might have allergies to specific foods.

So I went to this red book that the USDA had to see if I could somehow figure what I could "cook up" to check this out. I thought about Asia and how many thousands of years the people there lived on rice, soy, and vegetables. So I cooked up this brown rice, carrots, and celery with soybean loaf. At this time, Dr. Mark Morris, Sr., DVM, considered me the holistic veterinarian of California. He was the veterinarian who created Hill's Science Diets and that line of prescription animal foods. I sent my formula to Mark to see what he thought. He liked the diet and said to add a little calcium, which I did.

The diet had no name at this time but worked very well. Maybe this would be the future of not only creating a hypoallergenic diet but also a chance to build my bird-of-prey center. Everything was going well with my home made diet, until I heard from an irate husband who thought his wife was spending too many hours peeling carrots for the preparation of my diet for their dog.

His comment to me was, "If I have to watch my wife in the kitchen behind 5 feet of peeled carrots, I may have to kill you if you don't have your food produced commercially." I did get the message. I spoke with Hal Taylor from Breeders Choice and told him my predicament. I wanted to preserve the food without using preservatives. At the time, Breeders Choice was doing frozen loaves. I decided, if we used clean water, why not freeze the loaf? This is what happened. I called the frozen loaf Naturally Yours. It worked so well that wives would call me up and say, "You can't believe what happened. My husband came home late and decided to raid the refrigerator. He spied the loaf of Naturally Yours and devoured the entire loaf with Wheat Thins."

At the same time, I was finding that as many as 30 percent of my animals, and husbands, had food sensitivities. Soon an article came out of England, by a famous veterinary dermatologist, stating that less than 1 percent of dogs have food sensitivities. Life has been uphill since.

Soon thereafter, the son of a couple whose animals I had treated for many years came to me with a position. He had a ride foundation for handicapped children. He had received a bad batch of food from one of the local mills that had a weight-enhancing chemical for cattle called Mentensin. Apparently this is toxic in horses and destroys their livers. He found a trace mineral that has a liver-protective effect, which he felt saved half his horses. He asked me to research this trace mineral for a fee. I said I would be happy to do so for no charge, if he would help me develop a commercial, hypoallergenic diet. I spent one afternoon in his mother's home and designed Nature's Recipe. Eventually, after many years, the pets with hormonal imbalances became allergic to some of the ingredients. I then developed Innovative Veterinary Diets, with only one protein and one carbohydrate. As you know, many pet food manufacturers followed, which really did help clean up the pet food market.

I spent much time Friday afternoons at the UCLA Immunology Forum learning as much as I could to not only understand what was happening with my patients but also how to help them. At the time, Dr. Fayhe was kind enough to let me attend the forums even though I was a veterinarian. I am sure that the insights that I gained via the UCLA Medical Center have helped me find a better way to treat my veterinary patients.

[Dr. Plechner recently received an award from the American Veterinary Medical Association in recognition of his forty-four years of outstanding performance in the care of his patients.]

Curriculum Vitae

Dr. Alfred J. Plechner

September 2007

Education:

University of California, Los Angeles, Los Angeles, California

September 1956-1958

University of Southern California, Los Angeles, California

September 1958-1961

University of California, Davis School of Veterinary Medicine, Davis, California, Bachelor of Science & Doctor of Veterinary Medicine

June 1962

Background & Associations:

California Animal Hospital, Los Angeles, California

Partner and practicing veterinarian since 1968

Stonewood Meadows Wildlife Refuge, Calabasas, California Founder of state and federally licensed wildlife refuge specializing in the treatment and release of indigenous wildlife

Calabasas Cellars Vineyards & Winery, Calabasas, California Owner and operator, proceeds to fund wildlife refuge

Naturally Yours Pet Foods, Irwindale, California Creator of first non-meat commercial pet foods

Nature's Recipe Pet Foods/Earth Elements, Corona, California Creator of veterinary line of pet foods (IVD) Creator of consumer line of OTC pet foods (first Lamb & Rice) Consultant for research and development of other pet products

J.P. World Ltd., Malibu, California Research & formula consultant for product line (trace minerals, digestive enzymes, Omega 3 & 6, shampoos, and FoodGrownämultivitamins)

Big Horn Sheep Society of California, San Gabriel, California Research immunologist

A & E Laboratories Consultant for endocrine-immune blood work studies and general lab work

Association Memberships:

American Veterinary Medical Association

California Veterinary Medical Association

Southern California Veterinary Medical Association

Veterinary Allergy Academy

American Animal Hospital Association

American Holistic Veterinary Medical Association

Published Works:

Endocrine-Immune Mechanisms in Animals and Human Health Implications, A Compendium of Articles. Dr. Alfred J. Plechner, DVM, 2011

Curriculum Vitae

Contains:

"Unrecognized Endocrine-Immune Defects in Multiple Diseases"

"Adrenal-Immune Disturbance in Animals Offers Therapeutic

Insights for Multiple Human Disorders"

"Do Adrenal-Immune Disturbances in Animals and Common

Variable Immunodeficiency in Humans Have a Common Cause?"

"Cortisol Abnormality as a Cause of Elevated Estrogen and Immune Destabilization"

"Importance of IgA"

"Reproductive Failure and Adrenal-Thyroid-Immune Dysfunction"

"Adrenal Toxicity and Hormonal and Immune Destabilization in Animals"

"Innovative Cancer Therapy That Saves Animals, May Work For Humans"

"Suggested Human Protocol and Important Considerations"

"Blood Test and Evaluations"

"Therapy Possibilities for Humans"

Additional publications:

Pets at Risk, from Allergies to Cancer, Plechner and Zucker, New Sage Press, 2003

Pet Allergies, Remedies for an Epidemic, Plechner and Zucker, Very Healthy Enterprises, Los Angeles, California, 1986

"Skin Problems—Mineral Supplements May Be The Answer," *Pet Age*, November 1985, p. 24

"Canine Nutrition," *Pet Age*, February 1983, p. 20

"Feline Nutrition—Read The Label," *Pet Age*, February 1982, p. 12

"Preliminary Observations On Endocrine-Associated Immunodeficiency In Dogs—A Clinician Explores The Relationship of Immunodeficiency to Endocrinopathy," *Modern Veterinary Practice*, October 1979, p. 811

"Theory of Endocrine Immune Surveillance," *California Veterinarian*, January 1979, p. 12

"Endocrine Immune Surveillance," Plechner, Shannon, Epstein, Goldstein, and Howard, *Pulse*, June-July 1978

"Food Mediated Disorders," *California Veterinarian*, June 1978

"Food Induced Hypersensitivity," Plechner and Shannon, *Modern Veterinary Practice*, March 1977, p. 225

"Canine Immune Complex Diseases," Plechner and Shannon, *Modern Veterinary Practice*, November 1976, p. 917

Choosing the Right Pet for You and Your Family

Before you choose a special pet, you should check out available dogs and cats with local rescue groups and animal shelters. It is difficult not to bring home more than one animal. We have three dogs and three cats.

If you decide on a dog or cat, pick a breed that will fit the personality of the family. Abbys and Siamese cats love to vocalize. And many cats that are not purebred but have some of these breeds in them will often follow you around the house and talk to you. I happen to love this, but you may not. Many times they will want to be hugged and fondled. Again, if you want an animal that is less intense, possibly some sort of reptile might work. Remember, when you choose your pet, you need to realize that you have taken on a major responsibility. Your pet needs to be cared for in a manner in which you and your pet can flourish to a ripe old age. I have had a cat patient live to twenty-eight years of age and a dog patient live to twenty-seven years of age. Again, remember that this will hopefully be a long-term, happy investment for both you and your pet.

Let's talk about dogs. Do you want a laidback dog for you and the kids? Do you want a dog you can jog with? Most dogs can jog, but certain breeds are more readily adaptable for jogging. Do you want a dog for security? Often people will choose a breed that most criminals are afraid of. This is all good and fine, but most people who rescue or buy these animals are really not educated to train these dogs correctly. This is why you see the horrible stories about maulings of people, children, and other animals. Pit Bulls, Doberman Pinschers, and Rottweilers have been singled out as dangerous animals! The true dangerous animal happens to be the uneducated owner. Many people live their egos through their macho pets, since possibly they themselves are not. Remember this—there are no bad dogs, only bad owners. Think about it. Be the good person your dog or cat thinks you are.

I would like to tell you about an event that happened that shows the importance of picking the right pet for you and your family. A television program showed an unfortunate animal care officer approaching a house to check on a Pit Bull, and the owner came out of the front door and told Spike to attack the officer.

The dog did what the owner told him to do; he tore into this woman with no hesitation. Thankfully the animal care officer survived the attack. This had been filmed and shared on television all over our nation. Two days later, I was asked to appear on *Good Morning Los Angeles*. The panel on this program discussed the Pit Bull issue and came to the conclusion that there are only bad Pit Bull owners and not bad Pit Bulls. I recently watched an episode of *Dog Whisperer*, and Cesar Millan came to the same conclusion. After the *Good Morning Los Angeles* program, I went back to my practice. I was just checking on my patients to see if any of them needed anything. When one of my associates asked me to help him and give a quick rabies injection to a dog, I said I would, but normally I have an assistant to hold the patient for me while I give the injection. No one was available. I went to this dog, which was a beautiful, tricolored Pit Bull that was heavily muscled. He proceeded to jump up and lick me on the face. As I injected him, he kept licking me and wagging his tail. Just a gorgeous dog anyone would love to invite into his or her family. It turned out that this was the son of Spike, the dog that had raised havoc on television with the animal control officer because of the owner. This is one reason why you need to pick a pet that will fit you, your family, and also fit the pet.

If you choose a dog that needs to walk slowly, for example because of your arthritis, do not get a hunting breed. If you want to take your dog on walks in a protected area, do not get a field trial breed, as they have been trained to run long and be controlled only with a whistle, not an electric collar. In all fairness, putting a collar on a hunting dog or field trial dog is usually there for the dog's protection. Rule one of Dr. Plechner's rules for training your pet is that you must be smarter than your pet. Most people fail at this. If you really do not want to get involved in training your pet, a professional can do it for you. You may want to avoid terriers. They are outstanding dogs but definitely have a mind of their own and sometimes can be difficult to housebreak, particularly if you failed my rule number one.

There is often a classic mismatch of a wonderful family and a wonderful puppy. Often people will pick a puppy with great eyes, a unique color, or just a great look and personality. I, personally, have never seen a puppy that I would not take home with me. And trust me, I have taken all of my broken puppies home with me and fixed them or found great homes for them where, occasionally, I would be able to see them.

One family had just lost an older pet and decided that they needed to fill their house with happiness, and the sooner the better. So, they brought home Mabel, an eight-week-old Queensland Heeler. Oh, oh! She was so cute you could not believe it. Everything was great. She appeared to settle in with the family. However, she was bred to drive and guide herd animals by nipping at their heels. One evening, the family held a major party in Malibu and invited three hundred guests. An entire herd of people—you might imagine what happened next. Mabel lay under the couch and, to the horror of the hosts, she would race out and bite the back of the shoes of those guests who made the fatal mistake of getting near Mabel. It sounded to me like Mabel was not only doing a good job, but was doing exactly what she had been bred to do. She was now in a herd of people. The owners asked me to check Mabel to see if she had elevated total estrogen that might cause her behavior. Mabel was perfectly normal. It was apparent that Mabel did not fulfill the family's needs, and they did not fulfill hers. However, after a little behavior modification of the family, everyone lived happily ever after.

Hopefully, some of these ideas will make it easier for you to find a wonderful pet that not only will fulfill your needs, but whose needs you can also fulfill, and you can have a happy, long life together.

Pet Food

How do you determine if it is healthy for your pet?

Please realize, good foods for ourselves and pets are simple. Good nutrition is simple. The longer the label, the worse the food is, because good nutrition is simple.

Let's read the label.

How do we do this? It really is very simple.

The following facts will help you do this.

Please realize, 90 percent of the diet is explained and completed with the first three ingredients.

Are those ingredients protein or carbohydrates or both?

If beef or chicken or whatever is the fourth or fifth ingredient, this means the bull or the chicken came by the barn and waved. A diet that needs to have preservatives in it to guarantee that the diet is fresh and will not deteriorate before you feed it to your pet is very questionable.

Please avoid diets preserved with BHA, BHT, and Ethoxiquin. These preservatives may try to keep the color and longevity for that particular food, but why feed it to your pet?

Very simply, as you read the label, would you think the ingredients in the food would be worthwhile food for you or your child?

Often, the word *byproduct* means the diet is defective. You are correct if the byproduct is not defined by what it is labeled. Healthy byproducts do exist. What, then, really is the byproduct?

A byproduct can be a healthy form of protein that we as humans may not eat routinely.

A byproduct may mean a liver, lung, heart, or, in chickens and turkeys, a gizzard. These are fine, but what about unlisted or unnamed byproducts? What can those be, and are they healthy for you or your pet?

Have you ever realized that a chicken byproduct may mean feathers, feet, and wattles?

How about a beef byproduct? This can be hooves, hair, and horns. You probably don't want to take a chance on feeding an unnamed byproduct that might be harmful to your pet.

What about fiber? Almost immediately, you can tell if this is a cheap diet or not. Most cheap diets use beet pulp for fiber, whereas the better diets use tomato pumice. Beware of foods that contain peanut shells for fiber, as they can contain a type of fungal toxin that is lethal.

Let's talk about puppy and kitten foods. Would you feed your child more protein, carbohydrates, and fats? Of course not! So why would you do this to your puppy or kitten? This is merely an industry sales pitch to broaden food sales.

As you may guess, to use the feeding directions on the dog or cat food can or bag is ridiculous. If you put thirty children in a room for the day and feed them each three sandwiches for the day, some will gain weight, some will lose weight, and some will stay the same. If your pet is normal and can absorb nutrients normally, and your pet is producing more than three stools a day, you are feeding your pet too much.

Is your dog or cat overweight? The first thing to realize is that dry food (kibble) contains three times the calories of wet food. Does this give you a new idea as to feeding your pet, whether a dog or cat, in a different manner?

How about dry food and bones keeping your pet's teeth clean?

This makes as much sense as your dentist telling you to eat a hard English tea biscuit every day, and you would never need your teeth cleaned. It has never worked that way and never will. Dogs and cats are similar to their owners, and some people need to have their teeth cleaned three to four times a year because of a genetic imbalance, while other people never need to have their teeth cleaned even if they are not eating hard biscuits or kibble.

You need to realize that there is a better way, and try to not hurt your animal due to manufacturing concerns and misinformation designed to merely sell you products that could be detrimental to the health of your pet.

Please always read the label and decide if the product would likely be good for you before you feed it to your pet.

Foods That Contain Estrogen Inhibitors

The following is a list of foods that will help lower estrogen levels that may be too high in you or your animal. Hopefully this list will help you and your pet with elevated estrogen to become healthier.

- All kinds of berries

- Broccoli

- Buckwheat

- Cabbage

- Citrus fruits (grapefruit, oranges, lemons)

- Corn

- Figs

- Most fruits, except apples, cherries, dates, and pomegranates

- Grapes

- Green beans

- Melons

- Millet

- Onions

- Pineapple

- Squashes

- Tapioca

- White rice

- White flour

This is all good and fine and will give you an idea of which foods will be good for you and your pet if you have too much estrogen.

You need to also know, if you have gout, these foods may bind estrogen but also contain high levels of purines that can raise havoc with gout suffers.

Puppy Mills

For many years I've consistently tried to educate the general public on where to look when they want a new puppy and what they should check for to make sure the puppy does not come from a puppy mill. By now I'm sure most of you are aware that puppy mills churn out poor little creatures that have been designed to die early and painfully in life by "flesh peddlers" who don't care about the dogs or their new owners; they only care about the money that those dogs bring in. To puppy mill owners, dogs and their puppies are nothing but a cash crop. They have no emotion in what they do to make sure their crop is producing the most money they can get, including killing any dog that is damaged or that stops producing puppies in the quickest and most cost-efficient manner they can, usually by shooting them.

Can you imagine my feelings, almost twenty years ago now, in seeing a puppy mill puppy a small child was holding in his arms and, with his entire family's support, asking me to save the poor puppy? I could already tell that boy's puppy was so badly damaged genetically that there was no way that Mother Nature would let it live. It tore my heart apart when I had to deliver the bad news, and I vowed then and there to do something about it. And so began my quest.

I contacted a local news channel in Los Angeles, ABC Channel 7 News with Paul Moyer, and got them to do a five-night special series on the horror of puppy mills. From that series, we were able to get laws passed in the state stating that a puppy had to be eight weeks or older, with teeth, to be allowed to be shipped to California, and pet shops who sold puppies would be held responsible for all health problems that puppy might have for a certain amount of time after it was sold.

In my practice I offered all new puppy owners a free health exam, and if I found any problems I'd tell the puppy's owner and let them decide what to do with the pet shop. But though my efforts did put a dent in the puppy mills' profits in California and made some pet shops more responsible for the puppies they sold, the problem is as bad today as it was when I first started my quest.

And there is another, more sinister side of puppies that come out of puppy mills. A large majority of these dogs are genetically damaged because of the breeding methods of the flesh peddlers. Remember, they are in this only for the money and don't care if the animals that come from them are prone to cancer, allergies, seizures, and more. As long as the puppy is cute and as long as there is a pet store or owner willing to buy and pay them cash, they are in. And if you have a puppy mill dog, please have it fixed (spayed or neutered). The pleasure your child may get from seeing a dog birth puppies is not comparable to the sadness of taking unwanted puppies to the animal shelter where they will be put to sleep if no one adopts them.

I actually flew back to New York with some of my clients with genetically damaged pets and appeared on the *Geraldo* show. It still may be available. Geraldo had our side, the veterinarian, and the owners of the damaged pups they'd grown to love but were now suffering along with, and the puppy mill owners who, of course, protested all the way. And I had the opportunity to look into the eyes of these flesh peddlers and listen to how many "heads of dogs and cats" they sell. Dogs that wind up as part of a puppy mill operation are definitely God's most unhappy animals.

The battle of the puppy mill continues. The governmental agency that oversees them is understaffed, underfunded, and many times the staff just doesn't care. It is up to us to financially shut these people down (including our backyard local puppy mills—breeders who, on a smaller scale, are breeding puppies for the same motive and under the same squalid conditions as the larger scale puppy mills).

Here is what you can do:

- Never accept a puppy that does not have a forty-eight-hour return policy after your veterinarian has examined the puppy. If the puppy is returned, make sure in your original agreement that you will receive full compensation and not a replacement, also damaged, puppy.

- If you buy your puppy from a family, you not only need to have the same agreement as above, but meet the parents of the puppy. This will give you an idea of what your puppy will be like in adulthood.

If we all pay attention to some of these facts, many of the flesh peddlers will find it less feasible financially to carry on. The only way to stop these people while waiting for the authorities to get their act together is to hit the flesh peddlers in the pocketbook so that they cannot make a living creating poor helpless creatures that mean so much to the families who wind up losing them through an early prearranged death. Oprah had the right recommendation. Rather than buy a puppy from a pet store (she said 99 percent of puppies in pet stores come from puppy mills), go to your local animal shelter to adopt. Once you have an animal, unless you are planning on breeding it, have it spayed or neutered so that you are not accidentally contributing to the overpopulation of pets that wind up in shelters having to be euthanized.

Euthanasia

This is such a difficult subject to bridge!

There are so many questions to ask, when the time has come, when the procedure must be considered.

I do not have all the answers, but I do know when the recommendation needs to be made.

When your beloved pet goes from "living" to "existing," this is the time to respect his or her need to "transcend." None of us would want to not live life to its fullest, nor would we ever want to be in a position where we soil ourselves and can only experience the feelings of deterioration and suffering.

When the time has arrived, you need only think about your pet, not yourself. You need to remember the happy years your pet gave to you and respect your pet in his or her final days.

Often, you want to be with your pet when the euthanasia is done. What you need to remember is that your pet will sense your grief, and it may make the situation worse even though you mean well.

When I am in this situation professionally, I will usually give to my patient a large amount of tranquilizer and have the owner spend ten to fifteen minutes with the pet, until the pet is tranquilized. I think it is best for all at this time for the owners to leave and remember the pet as the pet would like to be remembered.

Just so you know what my feelings are, you need to realize I am about prevention and, after helping a patient live well for many years, having to do euthanasia is very difficult for me. I will hold my emotions in front of the owners, who are trying to do the same thing, but after I excuse myself, I find a private place where I can experience my grief without others seeing. No, I will never get used to doing this when my mission in life is only to heal.

When I was in active practice here in California, I would never charge a fee for euthanasia. I would rather see that money go to buying and caring for another pet. I did send in a donation to the Tree People in California to plant a tree for each animal, in that animal's name, in a state or national forest. In Asia, when a child is born or an old person dies, a tree is planted in his or her name. It gives the family a chance to walk through the forest of their loved ones.

The hardest thing in the world may be to have another dog or cat, but your deceased pet would want you to do this. You have an obligation to so many of the innocent animals that are being put to sleep every day because of overpopulation and lack of finances to give them a wonderful home. We are seeing so many precious animals taken to animal shelters because the owners cannot feed their pets, much less themselves and their children. Rescue groups are doing everything they can do to rescue these animals and place them in wonderful homes, but many of their rescues are being returned because people are losing their jobs and their homes. You not only need to make the difference to these animals but also to yourself because you will never again be able to experience the joy that an animal will give to you with unquestionable love and loyalty.

Yes, you must continue on, and I must as well.

I hope this section will give you the understanding you need to help both your pet and yourself at your pet's end of life.

Our beloved animals often are the only things that justify our lives.

Hints on How to Tell Who is Doing What in the Cat Box or in the Yard

Have you ever been faced with a multiple-pet household where one of the pets is doing something wrong or may have a problem that needs to be identified? Sometime you may find that one of your pets has tapeworms or round worms in his or her stool. Whose stool was it? One of the household pets has diarrhea. Possibly one of the pets happens to be eating a lot but losing weight? Is this pet not absorbing nutrients properly? You can tell this by the excess numbers of stools that are being produced. But, whose stool is it really? Who is defecating on the carpet or in the workout bag or in the new flowerbed?

This is simple to determine.

Merely buy a food dye from the market, and put it into the suspect's food. If you have no idea who is responsible for whatever, then put no dye in one food and different dyes in the other pets' food. Just keep track of the colors and who got each one.

If one pet is defecating on a white carpet, just make sure the stain from the dye is removable. The dye also may show in the urine.

It might be nice not to have to take in multiple stool samples and have to pay for each one.

I hope this hint will be helpful to both you and your veterinarian.

Flea Sensitivity

Fleas in general can be a major problem for people and their pets. Hopefully you have never experienced a flea infestation where your pets and you suffering from fleabites all over your bodies.

Normally, proper flea management can be provided for your pet by your health care professional.

There are monthly pills and applied liquids that can be used for flea deterrents. The newer monthly oral flea deterrents appear to be extremely efficient and much less toxic than the applied flea products, but, being a fairly new product, we are waiting to see what the long-term effects might be.

The application of some of these externally applied flea deterrent chemicals have caused some very serious side effects in both dogs and cats. In 2010, the EPA published a report on "spot on" applied flea chemicals that is quite disturbing. You should definitely Google their report before deciding which type of flea deterrent to use.

A great rule of thumb that has worked for me for over forty years has been, "If I would not apply this to myself, then why would I apply it to my pet?"

If your pet has allergies, autoimmunity, or cancer, remember that chemicals applied to the skin can traverse the skin, affect the internal organs, and worsen their original condition.

I have found, through my own clinical studies, that allergies, autoimmunity, and cancer all have a basis in hormone-antibody imbalances. If you believe that there is a need to identify this imbalance before applying a flea deterrent, please read about Plechner's Syndrome and how to control the imbalance first.

In a multiple-pet household, have you ever wondered why one pet has a flea attraction and the others pets do not? The answer is quite simple.

That particular animal may have a hormonal-antibody imbalance that can lead to a nutritional deficiency, which the fleas will sense. The fleas are sent by Mother Nature to destroy this animal because it either has a genetic defect or has acquired this defect through aging or possibly through toxins in the environment.

Obviously, flea control in general is still highly important, but if your pet, or just one of your pets, has a flea attraction, but you do not have an increased flea population where you and your pet live, this flea attraction might be solved by identifying this syndrome and replacing the altered hormones, returning to a normal immune regulation in the animal.

As you continue to read this book, you will begin to realize that many more serious problems can occur to your pet when there is an immune mechanism imbalance, besides just a "fleabite allergy."

Fleas normally live in the grass and feed on their host. Just because you have taken steps to control the flea problem in the house, this does not mean that your living quarters will be flea-free as a result. Until you control the flea population that lives in the grass in your yard, you may still have fleas in your house.

During an epidemic of fleas in your neighborhood, keep your pet off the streets and out of the dog park to help stop flea exposure to your pet and the spread of the fleas while walking or exercising your pet outside of your home.

Hopefully this information will help keep you, your family, and your pets free from a flea buildup and consequent fleabites!

Plechner's Syndrome Defined and Explained

Plechner's Syndrome is an accumulation of a widely varying group of clinical signs and symptoms that characterize any of a variety of disease abnormalities or conditions that create a specific identifiable pattern in specific hormone and antibody levels in blood serum of several species of mammals. This syndrome is due to a damaged middle layer adrenal cortex because of a genetic predisposition, environmental toxins, or aging. This damaged middle layer adrenal cortex in turn causes a reduction in active (working) cortisol, resulting in an elevated amount of estrogen to be produced by the inner layer adrenal cortex. Normal amounts of cortisol may be present; however, this cortisol can be defective or bound, and the same estrogenic effect may occur. The cortisol and estrogen imbalance usually presents itself as an altered immunity status with antibody depression present. This not only may result in malabsorption from the intestines, but also allows the immune cells to lose recognition of the body's own tissue and thus attack their own host. These changes in glandular performance allow for a variety of medical effects to occur, from allergies to irritable bowel disease, autoimmunity, uncontrolled tissue growth, and cancer.

Plechner's Syndrome (a typical cortisol imbalance syndrome) is simply a collection of clinical signs and symptoms that mimic a variety of disease irregularities or conditions in several species of mammals, including man. The presence of this syndrome is easily determined by a discernable and identifiable pattern in specific hormone and antibody levels in a simple blood serum test.

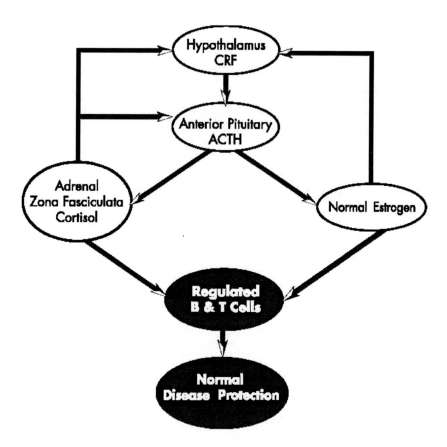

FIGURE 1: *This diagram shows normal relationships and feedback activity between the adrenal cortex and the hypothalamus and pituitary, and in turn, a healthy regulatory influence on the immune system.*

This syndrome gains access to the body through a glandular deficiency. The middle layer of the adrenal cortex becomes compromised because of aging, genetic susceptibility, environmental contamination, or possibly a combination of any of the above.

This impairment, in turn, causes a decrease in active (working) cortisol hormone, subsequently leading to an increase in the production of estrogen hormone by the inner layer of the adrenal cortex. Even though correct quantities of cortisol may, in fact, be available, the cortisol present may be defective or bound and not recognized by the pituitary gland, which in turn continues its production of its hormone (ACTH) and keeps requesting more active cortisol (which cannot happen) and only leads to the production of more excess adrenal estrogen.

This inequity of cortisol and adrenal estrogen causes an imbalance in the immune system and slows the production of antibodies. The results of these actions grow even more insidious. Not only do they negate the intestine's ability to absorb nutrients, medicines, and prescription drugs, but they also cause the immune cells (the body's protectors) to lose recognition of the body's own tissues, thereby canceling their protective function for the body and causing them to attack and cause damage to the body itself.

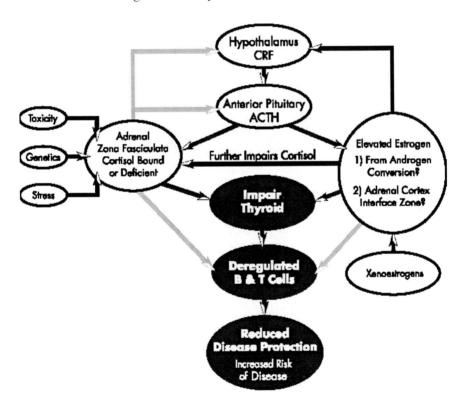

FIGURE 2. *Genetic and toxicity factors can interfere with cortisol production, triggering excess ACTH and estrogen release. Cortisol deficiency is aggravated, thyroid function affected, and the immune system destabilized.*

The effects of this rarely recognized syndrome may lead to a variety of ailments and diseases ranging from allergies and irritable bowel disease to autoimmunity, uncontrolled tissue growth, cancer, and other catastrophic diseases.

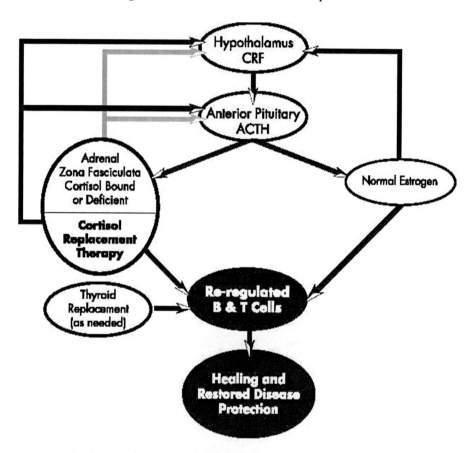

FIGURE 3: *Correction of cortisol deficit with cortisol replacement therapy restores normal hypothalamus-pituitary-adrenal relationships and immune system integrity. Thyroid replacement is typically required for canines, but not for felines.*

How to Determine if Exogenous Estrogen Mimickers Might be a Problem?

In today's world, measuring total endogenous estrogen, or estrogens produced by the body, may not be enough.

So far, the medical community does not realize that most of the estrogen that is produced in the body comes from the inner layer adrenal cortex in both males and females and is only partnered by a monthly estrogen input from the ovaries in females that are still ovulating.

Plechner's Syndrome explains why this elevated estrogen occurs and how to regulate its level to avoid allergies, autoimmunity, and cancer. What the medical community does not realize is that the total estrogen that is produced in the body will not measure the specific chemicals that are estrogen mimickers.

These estrogen mimickers include pesticides, plant estrogens called phytoestrogens, and those estrogen mimickers that come from plastics, referred to as xenoestrogens.

How, then, can you determine if you, your family, or pet are suffering from these estrogen-mimicking sources unless you test for a specific chemical or estrogen mimicker?

You really can't!

This is not financially practical or realistic, so it may be necessary to investigate the food you are eating and feeding and also try to realize if you, your family, or your family pet have been exposed to a chemical estrogen mimicker.

At this point in time, when doing this may not be realistic, why not test for Plechner's Syndrome to see if those estrogens produced within the body are normal or if there may be another input?

It has been proven that almost all these estrogen-mimicking chemical inhibitors do cause immune suppression of antibodies, and this is why Plechner's Syndrome should be tested for—to see if the total endogenous estrogens and other hormones are normal and if the measurable antibody levels (immunoglobulins) are suppressed, and, if they are, if there is good evidence that all of your family, including your pets, are being exposed to some sort of chemical estrogen mimickers.

Determining if a High Cortisol Value is Active or Bound

An overproduction of cortisol is called Cushing's Syndrome. But the real Cushing's Syndrome is an excess production of active cortisol produced by the middle layer of the adrenal cortex. Dr. Harvey Cushing identified a tumor in the pituitary gland that produced a hormone called ACTH, which caused the middle layer adrenal cortex to produce too much active cortisol. It is thought that a tumor of this middle layer adrenal cortex may also cause the production of too much active cortisol. It is also thought that giving too much cortisone can cause an increased production of active cortisone, which is true if the cells in the middle adrenal cortex are still productive, or this cannot happen. If these cells are still productive and exogenous steroids are given, this is referred to as iatrogenic, which means that the use of a cortisol replacement by your health care professional has caused this excess production of active cortisol. It is also thought that providing cortisone to a patient may lead to an inflammation of the pancreas, including the possibility of diabetes resulting. This has been proven wrong. It is the general belief by the veterinary profession that a cortisol replacement will cause diabetes mellitus in cats and may contribute to its development in dogs.

I do an endocrine immune test on each patient to determine if a cortisol imbalance is present before any cortisol replacement therapy is started.

In very few cases, when a diabetic state does occur, it appears to be a further extension of the original disease. If this does occur, the patient is successfully treated with the continuation of the cortisol replacement including the use of insulin. I found that stopping the cortisol replacement in order to regulate blood sugar level only often will lead to the demise of the patient.

How do you know if an elevated amount of cortisol is active or inactive? An elevated, empirical amount of cortisol does not guarantee that it will work in that patient. You may be told that the cortisol level is elevated, so it may be important to give the patient a chemical to reduce the amount of cortisol that is being produced from the middle layer adrenal cortex. These levels may be empirical and can only be proven viable by looking at those levels that active cortisol regulates. If these levels of high cortisol are bound or defective, the chemical given to reduce these high, but defective, levels may really hurt the patient.

Mere measurement of the empirical levels of cortisol alone will never be the answer to helping the patient. Even if your health care specialists do not relate to this, they can relate to the fact that a complete blood count (CBC) may show a deficiency in two types of white blood cells. Those deficiencies include a reduced number of lymphocytes and eosinophils. If these cells are present in normal numbers, this may be an inactive cortisol. If these cells are in a reduced state, the elevated volume of cortisol is probably active, and the use of chemical intervention may be indicated and of value. If this chemical is used in a patient that has high, inactive cortisol, this could cause that patient to lose his or her life.

It sounds like it is time to do comparative levels before the chemical treatment is prescribed. By including total estrogen with Plechner's Syndrome testing, this will give you much better insight as to whether the cortisol is active or inactive. If the total estrogen level is high, then the cortisol is inactive. If the total estrogen level is low, as well as the IgA, IgM, and IgG, then the high cortisol is active and may be a true indicator of Cushing's Syndrome. A cortisol stimulation test, if the cortisol is inactive, may be of little value in diagnosing while trying to diagnose Plechner's Syndrome.

Just because the laboratory indicates that there is an overabundance of cortisol does not mean the laboratory test is accurate. Also, are you clinically seeing actual signs of an increased, active cortisol?

What are the signs you might expect to see with an active excess of cortisol? You should see increased consumption of water and increased urination. There should be hair loss without inflammation and pruritis [itchiness]. Even though there may be calcification of the skin, this also occurs in other disorders outside of those with a high cortisol level or defective or bound cortisol. This can also occur with kidney disease, diabetes, irritable bowel syndrome, an IgA deficiency, a digestive enzyme deficiency, chronic intestinal parasites, and a diet too high in oil-based foods. Let's go from here.

Please check out all the above first, and if any of the above clinical syndromes are not involved, it is time to check if the high cortisol level is actually real. I have already indicated ways to determine this, but are there other things that can cause an elevated cortisol result that may be defective?

First of all, you need to guarantee that the serum sample is spun down and refrigerated immediately. The use of a temperature strip may be the thing of the future to make sure the sample arrives refrigerated. The laboratory needs to also keep all these samples refrigerated. It is common practice at many laboratories to leave samples out and to run them in batches. If this is done, all the testing for cortisol plus other hormones and antibodies may be abnormally high. Again, this may lead to the use of a chemical to reduce the "test results"-elevated cortisol, which have only *tested* high because the serum was improperly handled and reached room temperature or higher.

Why not do testing for Plechner's Syndrome and receive results that are comparative and not empirical?

If the blood sample is to be handled correctly, you need to send the sample to qualified laboratories; many laboratories have neither the staff nor equipment to guarantee you and your health care professional accurate results. Improper handling of the blood plus inaccurate results could lead to a catastrophe for either you or your pet.

It is very important to realize that even though there may be a large amount of inactive cortisol present, its presence may still cause clinical side effects. This is important to know because, if active cortisol is given, a lower dose of the exogenous cortisol might be used to reduce the possibilities of increased water consumption and increased urination.

If the IgA level is below fifty-eight in you or your pet, administration of an active cortisol will not be absorbed, and the problem will continue.

Please do not accept any cortisol level test results without considering the possibility that this test result presented to you or your physician might be due to testing faults that could lead to an inaccurate level present, which in turn could lead to treatments that could cause you or your pet fatal damage.

Recent evidence from prominent schools of veterinary medicine indicates that elevated levels of estrogen can mimic high active cortisol. What kind of cortisol replacement will be efficient for you and your pet or pets?

If you have tried homeopathic, holistic, and herbal replacement with little to no response, you must realize this layer of the adrenal gland may be permanently damaged and not merely fatigued. You need to realize that you cannot enhance the integrity of tissue that is permanently damaged. To give to you or your pet embryonic or adult remnants of the organs that produce these hormones is naive. These remnants are digested by the enzymes that are present and only enter the bloodstream as proteins and amino acids, not hormones! Western synthetics may be your only hope, but in the early phases, only through injections, not oral supplementation.

It is thought by the medical profession that on the water retention scale, hydrocortisone is a two, which is the highest, and prednisolone is a one. However, prednisone is preferred by most medical doctors. Interestingly enough, doctors are afraid that a cortisone supplement may cause liver damage, yet they still use prednisone, which needs to be converted in the liver, to prednisolone! Why? The use of methylprednisolone in dogs and in humans may provide the least water retention. Cats usually do very well on prednisolone. Horses seem to do best on thyroid hormone because their cortisol imbalances are often due to adrenal suppression that may be temporary or due to the use of feed with elevated levels of estrogen present. Different hays throughout the country may be to blame. I do not believe this is recognized just yet.

The importance of this section is: be aware, and do not fall into those tragedies that have occurred due to inaccurate laboratory results and an absence of realizing the difference between active and inactive cortisol.

Other hormones that occur in the body may also fall into this category. This is why salivary and twenty-four-hour urine tests have been developed. These tests may distinguish between free and bound hormones, but what is the guarantee that the receptor sites for the use of these active hormones are not blocked? There are no guarantees! You must observe the clinical signs and symptoms of your patient and decide the best way to heal that patient.

Obese Pets in America

Look around, and you'll most likely notice that obesity among our dogs and cats is increasing at an alarming rate.

While there may be several contributing factors to this problem, probably the two major causes are overfeeding and lack of exercise.

Before you even start any of this weight loss program, make sure your veterinarian has given your pet a clean bill of health. Since you are now reading this book, you are probably aware of Plechner's Syndrome. This in itself can cause weight gain with it having nothing to do with diet. The only way you can be sure that your pet is not hypothyroid is to make sure both thyroid hormones are at normal levels. You must check not only T3 and T4, but you have to also check total estrogen to make sure the thyroid hormones are not bound by excess estrogen in the bloodstream. Better yet, you may want to do an overall check on your pet and do a comprehensive endocrine-immune blood test.

Exercise

Often, people who live in apartments make sure their pets are walked regularly because they wish to make up for the animal's confinement during the day. People who have large yards sometimes assume their pet will roam the yard and self-exercise. However, this usually is not the case. For example, what about the pets raised on a farm? They usually spend most of their time sleeping on the back porch.

Food

Did you know that dry food and snack biscuits have three times the calories of canned food? Having dry food available all the time may be ill-advised for the health of your pet. Obviously, there are those circumstances where it can't be helped.

Often feeding directions will be printed on the dry-food bag. It will tell how much to feed per pound of body weight. This makes about as much sense as telling one hundred pet owners who each weigh one hundred fifty pounds to eat the same amount of food each day and they will maintain their proper weight. Good luck! Unlike many human foods, there may not be facts on how many calories are contained in a cup of food. As with us, for pets, eating multiple small meals through the day is best. Eating one large meal per day might be contributing to all of our problems. If dry food has to be given, then only feed it in the morning and hope that the excess calories will be worked off before bedtime. For many years it was believed that to feed your pet from the leftover food from the table was a no-no. It might have been if the owners were not eating correctly themselves! Realistically, while avoiding highly seasoned foods, most salads, pastas, fresh or steamed vegetables, and fruit are high in nutrients, vitamins, and enzymes, and are very acceptable when added to our pet's base food. If you are so inclined to reduce the amount of dry food only, it is very easy to cook up a vegetable stew and add this to the dry base food, which should satisfy your pet's hunger.

Cats definitely have more specific tastes than dogs. If they will eat more canned food and less dry food, this will help reduce their weight. If the cat will eat only dry food, then try to cut down on the kibble and either mix into the dry food some of their favorite fresh protein, like chicken or fish, or add a little protein in the form of a baby food.

Snacks can really add on weight, even if the amount of protein is high in proportion to total calories. It can be simply too much in terms of total calorie intake. See if the pet might accept celery and carrots, which you can flavor with a little canned food, a tiny amount of peanut butter, or cheese. Cats often like small amounts of their favorite proteins. If all else fails, you can always use a small amount of their favorite kind of dry food, but only a very, very small amount.

How do you check your pet for obesity? Just observe your pet. From the side view, is there a sagging belly? Remember, this can be a dog or cat. From the top view, is there a waistline present behind the ribs? Is the collar, in the adult pet, tight, or has it had to be replaced in the last six months? Now lay your hands on your pet. First, run your hands along the ribs and see if you can even feel the ribs. If the ribs are not very prominent, carefully use your thumb and index finger and lightly pinch the tissue lying over the ribs. You can also do the same procedure in the tissue of the neck. If there is more than one-half inch between your fingers, for a dog, this will indicate too much "table muscle." Cats seem not to accumulate that much fat under their skin. A walk-on scale, if available, might be of value.

Realize that an overweight pet with a heart problem, arthritis, bad back, or bad knees and joints will only get worse and, with less exercise to burn off calories, will reach a point of not walking. Never decide to have a set distance for your pet to walk. Always watch and listen to your pet and when he or she begins to verbalize, limp, or just sit down, you have taken your pet too far. Short walks, long walks, and swimming are the best exercise for both you and your pet. The length of the walk needs to be decided by you and your pet. Remember this: no "weekend warrior" stuff! I have a friend, Joe Merlino, who is a physical fitness trainer. I have not spoken to Joe for a long time. He ran a wonderful pit bull rescue, and to get some of these dogs into a healthier physical shape, he ran them on his treadmill. I definitely do not want you to try this with yours. We will figure out a safer way for your pet to lose weight. We can leave dogs on treadmills for the professionals.

For those of you who live in mild or warm climates, especially during summer, you may want to think about reducing the amount of hair that your pet has. This is especially true for long-haired pets. Unfortunately, our pets normally only have functional sweat glands between their toes, and the majority of their bodies' excess heat is dissipated through respiration. By keeping your pet's temperature at a comfortable level, there is a better chance of burning off calories. Often, during these hot phases of weather, add ice cubes to your pet's water or replace the water with straight ice cubes. Never allow your pet at any time to rapidly drink large quantities of water. It is much safer to use ice cubes, and as they melt, this will allow your pet to drink water but only in small amounts at a time. The reason for slowing the animal's rapid intake is to avoid over hydration which can cause vomiting of the water. This can lead to an electrolyte imbalance which can be very disabling unless recognized and promptly treated.

Your Pet's Thyroid Gland

In both dogs and cats, there are two glands that lie in the neck just under the Adam's apple on either side. Knowing their location will help you check for any nodules or enlargements, often before clinical signs develop. Definitely have your veterinarian teach you how to check this gland. The actual theme of the book is to identify and correct any medical health problems before permanent damage occurs.

An enlargement of the thyroid gland is often referred to as a goiter. This condition may occur with either decreased or increased thyroid function.

The anatomical structure of the gland consists of outer follicles. These follicles are made up of cells that surround a center filled with a jellylike substance called colloid. The follicles produce two types of thyroid hormone into the bloodstream. One type of hormone is called T4, which is a reserve or "storage" hormone that can be converted into the second hormone, called T3. T3 is the active hormone that is used to control the metabolism in your pet's body. These hormones require iodine, which is obtained from the soil that edible plants are grown in. The soil around the Great Lakes has been called the Goiter Belt because of a lack of iodine in the soil. Many people, and probably pets, had enlarged thyroid glands due to deficiencies of iodine. Interestingly enough, in the late 1930s, Morton Salt Company began to iodize its salt product in order to counteract this iodine deficiency.

What is the actual function of the thyroid gland and its hormones? Its main function, in both you and your pet, is to regulate the glands and other tissues in the body and make sure they can perform in a manner conducive to good health in both. It determines how quickly the cells in the body utilize oxygen and how much waste product needs to be detoxified. These functions can be totally increased or slowed down according to thyroid function. In any event, the deregulated thyroid can cause some amazing disorders in you and your pet.

If there is a thyroid imbalance in your puppy, often there is not only a reduction in the development of the puppy, but personality problems may also occur. Current thinking is that the thyroid-stimulating hormone (TSH) from the pituitary gland controls the thyroid gland. What often is not realized is that there are many more inputs to the thyroid gland that can cause adversities.

Apparently, fluoride in our water supply does inhibit thyroid function. How does that affect your pet's thyroid? The use of soybeans and soybean oil can also disrupt thyroid function. It is thought that the fermented forms of soy, such as tofu and tempeh are okay, but I worry. Is there a form of estrogen in these products also? I personally try to avoid these products for my pets.

It was found in the 1940s that hog lard was a huge commodity, along with the price of their meat. Apparently, by feeding corn and soybeans to the hogs, there occurred a suppression of the thyroid, resulting in a larger fat production. I know some people have pigs as pets, so there is a need to feed them properly, but what happens to our dogs and cats when their food contains corn and soybeans? Realize that if your pets are allergic to wheat glutens, then corn and rice are two carbohydrates that do not contain glutens. It is interesting to think Siamese cats once guarded large stacks of corn to stop the rodents from eating it, and now modern-day man is including corn in their cats' diets. The world has really changed. I remember when I spent summers working for the Seaside Clam Company. The bait I used to catch salmon and sea perch is now being eaten in fancy restaurants as appetizers. How did that happen?

As you are beginning to understand, there are many factors that can derail a thyroid gland and its hormones. Besides the already mentioned deregulating factors, what else might cause a deficiency to occur? We have already discussed the mechanism.

- When the natural cortisol is deficient, bound, or not hydroxylated correctly, T4 thyroid hormone will not be properly transferred into T3, which is the active thyroid hormone, thus causing a thyroid deficiency.

- When the cortisol is imbalanced and is unable to fund the negative feedback mechanism to the pituitary gland, the pituitary gland then releases its hormone, ACTH, to ensure that more active cortisol will be released in order to maintain proper hormone balance. Since the middle layer adrenal cortex cannot respond, the inner layer takes over the response. This layer not only releases estrogen but also releases male hormones called androgens [DHEA and DHEAS]. In people, there is an enzyme in the fatty tissue, called aromatase, that turns not only female androgen into estrogen but also turns male testosterone into estrogen. What does this do? The high total estrogen not only binds the cortisol, but it also binds T3 and T4, therefore causing a further thyroid deficiency.

The high total estrogen also appears to deregulate the immune system, now allowing these essential cells to malfunction.

Not only do the immune cells cease to provide protection for the body, but it gives them a chance to lose recognition of "self" tissue. The only deficiency that occurs is in the B-cell production of antibody. When the antibody meant to protect the mucous membranes of the body drops below a certain level, malabsorption occurs. This antibody is referred to as IgA. If this is happening, do you think nutrients can be absorbed? Definitely not. Again, this is another reason the thyroid cannot feed itself and make proper hormones. Since the high total estrogen has created this state, the estrogen protects itself by reducing the metabolism of the liver and kidneys, where not only does breakdown occur, but excretion through the kidneys as well. The vicious cycle continues. Go ahead and give all the oral supplements in the world. With the high total free estrogen causing malabsorption, do you really think nutriceuticals, foods, and replacement hormones will be properly absorbed and make a difference? Not really.

Why not consider all of this and realize that you need to test this endocrine-immune mechanism to make sure that there is not a mechanism imbalance present? If there is, nothing given orally will be absorbed properly. Also, trying to enhance the integrity of glandular material is understandable, but you have to realize that you cannot enhance the integrity of something that is not there.

What Pet Owners Today Need to Know About Vaccinations

What is a vaccination? A vaccination is an injection of a virus, bacteria, or rickettsia in a solution. The microorganisms in the vaccine are either killed or modified live. In the live vaccine, the organism has been changed in a way that cannot cause a disease when injected. This modification process is called attenuation, and this process will allow the body to produce protective antibodies to that organism. In the future, when the patient with the protective antibodies is exposed to one of these diseases, the body will be protected. The first reported vaccine was the smallpox vaccine.

There are a great number of concerns that pet owners have regarding vaccinations. At the top of the list is, "Should I vaccinate my pet or not?"

The American Animal Hospital Association has updated information on the most recent thoughts about the proper way to administer vaccines. You can visit their website online to read more and also to obtain important contact information.

The modern thinking about vaccinations has experienced some major changes in the past few years. In my first practice, I used to check levels of protective antibodies that vaccines produced. I still vaccinate annually to somewhat guarantee that my patients all had enough protective immunity; however, our veterinary researchers have since found that protective antibody levels may remain high for three to seven years and in some up to ten to twelve years.

So why vaccinate at all? Young animals need to be safely introduced to disease vaccines at an early age. It is probably best to begin the vaccines at eight weeks of age. This is because the maternal antibodies that mom passed on to her offspring usually have disappeared at about this time. Maternal antibodies are usually present up to eight weeks and, if vaccinated before this time, will kill the modified live virus vaccine and create very little protective antibodies, if any at all. The feeling is somewhat the same for killed vaccines. Apparently there is very little protection achieved. The interval between giving vaccines may vary from veterinarian to veterinarian, but in our hospital, I recommend a vaccination at eight, twelve, and sixteen weeks of age for both puppies and kittens. In older dogs and cats with questionable vaccine histories, two vaccines at a one-month interval should suffice. Annual vaccines are usually recommended, but knowing the information already presented, annual vaccines may be a thing of the past. The question now is, if this is true, and the owners are very concerned about vaccination, why do them?

Can vaccines be detrimental? Yes, they can be. I have seen many reactions over the years. These reactions did not occur in my patients because I often checked current protective antibody levels in my patients prior to additional vaccinations. Because I have a special interest in allergy and hormonal antibody disorders, I have always been very conservative with the use of vaccines or any substance injected into the body. Sometimes we forget that each patient is different, whether an animal or a human. What might work for one might be detrimental to another.

There has been great controversy as far as the amount or volume of the vaccine to give. Often the same amount or volume of vaccine is given to a three-pound dog as to a two-hundred-pound dog. The manufacturers of the vaccine say a full dose is safe to give to any size dog because it is not the volume of the vaccine, but rather the "minimum immunizing dose."

Can you imagine the reaction that might occur with one vaccine? And what if more than one type of vaccine is given to this patient at the same time?

I have seen so many horrible reactions over the years that I have always used reduced volumes in my small patients and have successfully created proper immunity. Proper immunity was easily determined by doing a protective antibody level test two weeks after the primary vaccine program was completed. Recent thinking says, however, that a reduced vaccine dose will not create enough protective antibodies. Personally, I would rather give the smaller vaccine volume, check the antibody levels two weeks later for those vaccines that were administered, and if necessary give another vaccine two weeks later to avoid a possible reaction. A protective immunity that has been created through a vaccination procedure is referred to as an antibody titer. Doing antibody titers testing may be an extra expense, but it is much safer. You need to decide if your best friend is worth it or not.

A word about nosodes. This is a preparation that is sometimes used in place of present-day vaccines. Nosodes are used by holistic veterinarians and other veterinarians who are fearful of actual vaccinations being detrimental to their patients. In the hands of some veterinarians, the nosodes seem to work well. If they are getting protection for their patients, great, but in my hands, I was never able to create protective antibodies in my patients. I did check protective antibody levels [titers] after using this method and found a lack of protection. I have been told by other veterinarians that nosodes work in a different manner. However, I never pursued the issue because I saw several litters that had received nosodes and perished from contact with the various diseases that nosodes were used to protect against.

In all fairness, if the litters had my immune mechanism defect (endocrine-immune disorder), I am not sure anything would have worked, including vaccinations.

Many years ago, when people were afraid that the altered viruses and bacteria (attenuated) that were in the vaccines might still give the puppy distemper, a measles vaccine was developed.

The thinking was, in using the measles virus, it was close enough to the structure of the distemper virus that immunity would be created without the puppy getting distemper from this vaccine. Unfortunately, this did not happen. Later an altered distemper virus was added to the measles vaccine. I am really not sure why they kept including the measles virus; this virus was close enough to the structure of the distemper virus, but the general thinking was that the combination would be safer to use for annual vaccinations. That vaccine has since disappeared, and I think you can now begin to understand some of the controversy that has accompanied vaccinations for many years. I again refer you to the AAHA website for the most recent updates involving vaccine procedures.

It is important to know that the different vaccines must never be given in the same injection site. Also, from my standpoint, it is helpful to inject each specific vaccine into a different site on the patient. This means injecting the same vaccine in the same area every time in each patient. Different vaccines must never be given in the same injection site. This may lead to development of an incurable cancer called an injection site sarcoma. Performing this method of injections will help determine which vaccine caused the reaction, if any reaction does occur. Remember, each patient is different, and each patient may or may not react to one or many of the varieties of vaccines. Obviously, this information is important for both the owner and the veterinarian.

I favor giving vaccines in the lower lumbar area. This is the area just above the tail on either side of the spinal column. I do this mainly because if there is a reaction, it will occur higher on the back and not in the leg area, which may lead to motility impairment. Also, if the patient suddenly moves, there is no sciatic nerve to pierce. I have seen patients where this has happened, and permanent lameness remained for the life of the patient. And finally, for the patient's comfort when receiving any kind of injection, pat the patient firmly on the head while your veterinarian pinches the skin at the same time before introducing the needle into the patient. The patient's sensory center will be occupied, and the injection should be less painful. This is why many dentists, when injecting the patient with a local anesthetic, will lightly pinch and shake the cheek to occupy the sensory center.

My greatest concern is not so much with the use of vaccines, but rather with identifying the patients that will not stimulate the development of protective antibodies through vaccination. In the case studies section, I discuss a family that had vaccinated their pet properly and revaccinated many times to ensure their pet would remain healthy. What happened? At eighteen months of age, their dog contracted parvovirus and died.

The family then rescued a beautiful Harlequin Great Dane. The new owners wanted a guarantee that this would not happen again to their new puppy, but obviously there are no guarantees in medicine.

I have researched and have been able to create a test that will tell you whether your pet will have the ability to produce protective antibodies through vaccination. When there is a cortisol imbalance (this is a natural hormone that is produced in the middle layer adrenal cortex in both people and animals), Plechner's Syndrome may be indicated. When this hormone is deficient, bound, or defective, that layer may not be able to respond to the demands of a higher-up gland called the pituitary. Even though the pituitary gland is asking the middle layer for some more cortisol to carry out its job, the middle layer cannot respond. The only other layer in the body that can respond to the pituitary's demand is the inner layer of the adrenal cortex. This layer contains and produces a female hormone (estrogen) and a male hormone called androgen. When the estrogen level increases due to this imbalance, the higher amount of estrogen binds the thyroid hormones (thyroid hormones regulate metabolism throughout the body), which in turn somewhat protects the excess estrogen to let it remain while more is being produced. This is part of the vicious cycle that exists in Plechner's Syndrome patients. Furthermore, the higher-than-normal estrogen deregulates the two main types of immune cells that, when properly regulated, will protect the person or the animal. The one cell is called a B lymphocyte. Its function is to protect the body from bacterial infections and produce protective antibodies to foreign substances and vaccinations. With its deregulation caused by the high estrogen, the B cell not only does not protect the body from bacterial infections, but also does not produce antibodies to foreign materials and vaccinations. You can now hopefully see why the eighteen-month-old dog died from parvovirus after being vaccinated several times. She had Plechner's Syndrome.

Also, when the antibody in the stomach and intestines is deficient, then malabsorption occurs (the inability of nutrients and medications to pass into the patient's bloodstream). This is another part of the vicious cycle. Oral foods, nutriceuticals, and homeopathics, no matter how natural they may be, may not be able to reach the body through the bloodstream by way of the intestines. Hopefully you can now see why changing drugs and nutrients might be a waste of time. A prime example of this is when a patient is in the hospital on intravenous fluid and intramuscular injections, which bypass the intestines and go directly into the bloodstream, and they are effective. When the patient with Plechner's Syndrome is sent home on the same medicine in an oral form, they do poorly because of the low antibody level in the intestines and the inability to absorb. The T lymphocyte, when properly regulated by the hormones, protects the patient from viruses, mold, and fungi. When Plechner's Syndrome has occurred, the patient can suffer from multiple colds, flu, plus develop all kinds of allergies to different molds and fungi. Ongoing *Candida* infections (this is a yeast-like fungus that is normally in the mouth, intestines, and vagina in healthy people) are prevalent in people with Plechner's Syndrome. With the immune regulatory mechanism breakdown that occurs, the T cell will not protect the body, and rampant growth may occur. This also applies to increased growth of demodectic mange mites, which are normally present in the skin of dogs and the nasal tissue of some people, but only cause disease when Plechner's Syndrome has developed. It is important to realize that the B and T cell function, when reduced, can only lead to disease problems in those patients that have this syndrome. This loss of immune function may lead to loss of recognition of self tissue and can lead to autoimmunity and cancer.

It is important to realize that when this hormone imbalance occurs, both the B and T cells are deregulated and not only lose sight of self breakdown tissue but may react adversely to any foreign substance that invades the body. The fact that the B cell is not providing proper antibody does not mean that its entire function is depressed. It definitely is not. This is the mechanism that is the cause of allergies, autoimmunity, and cancer.

Hopefully this will give you some insight as how to vaccinate this new Great Dane puppy. First, the puppy was vaccinated at eight and then twelve weeks. Two weeks later I did a blood test to measure the level of the protective antibody (titer). Both levels of antibody protection for parvovirus and distemper were nearly nonexistent. I immediately did my hormone antibody panel. The results of the test indicated the following: low cortisol, high estrogen, a normal T3 and T4, but bound because of the high estrogen, and low antibody production. The antibody in her gut was high enough to allow for absorption of oral replacement hormones, so she was put on a cortisol and a thyroid replacement. In four weeks, her hormone antibody levels returned to normal, and her B cell now was ready to produce protective antibodies. During this replacement period, I cautioned the owners not to take the puppy out of their yard and house since the puppy had no protective immunity. I revaccinated the puppy at the same time interval as before, and two weeks past her last vaccination, I rechecked her protective antibody levels and found that the B cell had been reregulated by proper hormone replacement and now allowed to function in a protective manner.

Now the puppy has very high levels of protective antibodies to not only parvovirus and the distemper virus but also any other invasive organisms that B and T cells can neutralize.

With all the commentary on do or do not revaccinate, what should you do? After the initial vaccination program is completed, two weeks later, you should have your veterinarian test to see if your young animal has developed protective antibodies (titers). If your animal has not developed pro immunity, it might be worthwhile to give one more vaccine to see if this boosts the immunity to a protective level. If the vaccine did not help, then it is time to run an Endocrine Immune Panel 1 blood test. If the results are positive for Plechner's Syndrome, fund the patient's imbalance and then revaccinate. At this point in time, there is only one veterinary laboratory doing my blood test.

The details of how to handle the sample and where to send the sample are listed on my website at http://www.drplechner.com .

Please know, I have no affiliation with this laboratory, but no other labs have had much of an interest, and those labs that have looked into running these tests apparently do not have the equipment or the ability to reliably run these tests. This lab can do Endocrine Immune Panel 1 testing for dogs, cats, horses, and people.

One huge concern of the general public is what kind of chemicals, additives, and other ingredients go into the vaccines. Is it really the vaccine that is the problem, or is it the other ingredients that are added? The same danger is still there. Should the vaccines be "cleaned up," or are we still exposing ourselves, our pets, and our children to a needless danger?

Years ago, I found that a certain number of miniature poodles had severe reactions to vaccines. I also found that many of these patients were allergic to chicken egg embryo. Guess what the vaccines were created with? Yes, chicken egg embryo was the medium for growing the viruses. To say it is okay to vaccinate your child or animal with present-day vaccines is very questionable. How much of the attenuated virus, whether dead or modified live, is enough, and is not too much? How can we tell what has happened? The time has come when vaccine manufacturers need to take heed and research the problems that they may be causing. Also, remember that the problem may not be caused by the vaccine, but by an imbalance in the patient that allows the vaccine to cause negative effects, including no antibody protection.

Hopefully this information raises some very important thoughts for you to consider for yourself, your child, and your pet.

Impact Areas

Have you ever wondered why certain disorders occur in certain areas in the body?

What may be the reason?

So many disorders seem to randomly occur, but we really have no idea why. We have considered the effects of Plechner's Syndrome but have not really associated why they happen due to Plechner's Syndrome in specific organs or tissues in a given animal. Why, then, does one ear or eye always seem to be involved? Could this be because of an allergic reaction caused by Plechner's Syndrome?

Let's examine some things to see if there may be a reason. What things could cause this to occur? Many times there are more mast cells in one area then another. Mast cells contain histamine, which, when released, can cause a local inflammation in the nearby tissues. This is why one ear may chronically be inflamed if there are more mast cells in one area as opposed to another area.

Obviously, genetics must be involved, but what else could be an underlying cause? We know the environment can be involved, as well as age, anesthesia, vaccines, diet, nutrient availability, immune health, foodborne chemicals, genetically modified foods, and chemotherapy. So how do we stand on these issues, and how do we decide how to help the patient and not just accept the situation?

Without repeating myself, I suggest running the endocrine-immune blood test. You do not have to act upon the results, but for the benefit of your patient, you should pay attention to the facts that the test produced. If you are unable to do this for the patient's well-being, please refer the case to a veterinarian who is willing to make use of the hormone-balancing protocols to restore the proper balance in the patient's endocrine system.

With Plechner's Syndrome, we must realize that the high total estrogen is going to not only bind thyroid hormones but will also deregulate the immune system and will cause antibody protection to decrease. What does this really mean? It means that there are a large number of undesirable medical events that will occur. Think about this. If the regulatory mechanism of the endocrine system is defective and antibodies are deficient when you or your animal is vaccinated, no protective antibodies can be produced due to the imbalance. How many pets have died from preventable diseases even though they had received a specific vaccine for that disease?

Many diseases are thought to have been eradicated, yet with third-world children migrating into our country with less than proper medical care, we are again seeing diseases that we have been told are gone. What about our puppies and kittens? With this endocrine imbalance mechanism breakdown that we have talked about, do you really think our animals can make protective antibodies to these preventable diseases? Definitely not! Why even vaccinate an animal or a person who has this imbalance? The imbalanced individual most likely will not produce a protective level of the desired antibodies. I suspect that the vaccine antigens may even predispose the patient to developing catastrophic disorders, like autoimmune disease.

There is no way a patient whether human or animal can produce proper protective antibodies. When this vaccine, which is made of foreign protein, is administered to a patient, when the patient suffers from Plechner's Syndrome, this foreign protein cannot be properly processed and can lead to a catastrophic reaction without production of any protective antibodies.

You need to test for Plechner's Syndrome before you vaccinate. And if you do vaccinate, be sure to check the patient at twelve to sixteen weeks of age to see if the vaccine did create the desired protective antibodies. If the test doesn't show protective antibody levels, then you have missed Plechner's Syndrome. Recheck the hormone levels and do the hormone replacement and revaccinate at the appropriate time. I know many of you no longer vaccinate your young animals. This may be fine, but please be very careful that you are not putting your pet in danger.

Where else, then, do we see diseases due to Plechner's Syndrome? When the high total estrogen not only binds thyroid hormone but also causes the B cell lymphocyte to reduce its antibody production, what happens?

The B cell produces three main antibodies. The IgM is a primitive antibody that sharks have. This is kind of a roadblock antibody that first stops the foreign invader from hurting the body. Once this roadblock has performed its function then the IgG antibody makes antibodies specific to the invader. The IgA antibody is there to protect the mucous membranes of the body. Hopefully, now you have an idea where the disorder may occur. If the IgA imbalance has a genetic influence, this may determine where in the body the impact will be. So you tell me where the patient is going to be hit with a disease? Obviously, the disease will affect the mucous membranes of the body. Let me then give you some choices. Your pet could have an imbalance in his or her gums leading to gingivitis, in the digestive tract resulting in irritable bowel syndrome, or a respiratory disorder such as asthma. Or your pet could have ongoing kidney or urinary bladder issues. What about the genital tract? False pregnancy indicators will always be an issue, as well as infertility problems. There are definitely many other reasons why infertility occurs besides hypothyroidism unless the high total estrogen has bound the thyroid hormones. Trust me, it will take more than thyroid hormone to help this patient.

Have you ever been told that your dog or cat, because of his or her horrible gumline infection, needs to have all the teeth pulled to avoid more serious problems? Never, ever do this without first checking the IgA levels to make sure this is not a correctable situation. Why would you put your pet through this radical procedure without getting a second opinion? If you would not let someone extract all of your teeth, I suggest that you should not do it for your pet unless it is absolutely necessary.

Hopefully this will help you realize why our pets develop disorders in specific areas, and hopefully it has also given you some insight as to how to identify Plechner's Syndrome and control the problems.

Rage

This is a syndrome that has been seen in dogs, cats, horses, and probably people for many years.

It really is not known why this happens, but over the last forty-four years of practice, I have found a way to not only identify this syndrome but also to control it. I think we all wonder how this can occur and what really does occur during a rage.

Having a show dog growl or bite a judge to having a puppy bite your child or another family member is similar to the cat that decides its owner is worth biting or scratching. Why does this happen? I sometimes wonder if this might also explain road rage. Whether it does or not, there appears to be a way to identify and control the problem.

Many years ago, I was working with a friend and animal trainer, Michael Chill. The situation involved a Labrador retriever that, unprovoked, would attack the wife and the daughter. At this time, I was looking at the possibility of a food setting off this bizarre behavior. At this time, I had created the first lamb and rice diet in the country, if not the world. My friend decided to put the dog on lamb and rice to see if it would make a difference, and it did. The dog did very well, with no further episodes of rage.

Later, one Thursday evening, the family had a nice steak dinner and saved a small amount for their dog. Within thirty minutes, the dog attacked the wife severely enough that she had to go to emergency care.

Since then I have learned that a different food, a supplement, or a snack can elicit this vicious behavior. Why would this food input cause this effect?

After many years of my own clinical studies, I finally realized that Plechner's Syndrome was the culprit that allowed for the "rage syndrome" that I was seeing. I have been able to diagnose the disorder in patients and have had good success with calming rages through treatment of their Plechner's Syndrome.

Chronic Diseases in Pets

This defective regulatory mechanism has rarely been considered as the primary basis for many chronic diseases in pets. Plechner's Syndrome is actually a very simple hormonal regulatory mechanism, which has never before been identified. Nor have the results of serum hormone level tests been used to treat chronic diseases in pets and people. If all other medical diagnostic and treatment options have been tried and the disorder continues, why not at least have the tests done and see if this might be the basis for your pet's chronic liver problems, kidney and bladder problems, pancreatic problems, ongoing mange, ongoing skin problems, chronic reactions to yeast and fungi or mold, and more?

If you are a health care professional and you are getting good results with your diagnosis and treatment program, then good job. However, if you are not getting the results you want, you may just want to do this simple blood test to see if your patient has the hormonal imbalances that fit a diagnosis of Plechner's Syndrome. If your patient does have Plechner's Syndrome, I am more than happy to consult with you on the phone or via e-mail. There are many veterinarians and physicians using what I have learned who are bringing relief to their patients afflicted with chronic, often catastrophic, diseases. I promise you that until everything is known about all diseases, I will continue my quest to identify the causes of these diseases. I will continue my quest until I die.

Osteoporosis

My senior project at the University of California at the Davis School of Veterinary Medicine was working with a wonderful cougar cub named Tigger.

He jumped off of a small step and fractured his front legs. His symptoms were compared to those of a genetic disease called Osteogenesis imperfecta.

With my consequent studies, I found that a nutritional problem really caused Tigger's problem. At this same time, the zoos continued to feed their captive big cats a straight meat diet, and they were seeing the same problems that Tigger had in their big cats.

The reason this was happening was because a straight meat diet—without bones—provides one part calcium and twenty parts phosphorous.

The body, whether Tigger's, yours, mine, or the large zoo cats', tries to keep a one-to-one or one-to-two ratio between calcium and phosphorus, and when only raw meat is used to feed these animals, the improper ratio continues to exist in their nutritional status.

In order to reestablish the normal ratio of calcium and phosphorus, the body will remove nineteen molecules of calcium from the animal's bones to match the twenty molecules of phosphorous.

You can begin to see how this will affect our pets and our own bodies.

Soon after realizing this, I developed a balanced diet for dogs and cats; a few years later my formulation was modified slightly for zoo cats. As I remember, it was called ZooPreme. After eating this balanced mineral diet, their osteoporosis problems disappeared.

At this same time, Siamese kittens were suffering from the same mineral imbalance. They would jump off of a step and fracture one or both of their front legs. By adding proper amounts of calcium to their food, the problem did not occur.

What other bone loss diseases do we see based upon this ratio? We see chronic kidney disease that can increase retention of phosphorous, which causes calcium to be removed from the bones in animals and their owners.

We also see Plechner's Syndrome in pets and their owners. When an adrenal imbalance causes excess adrenal estrogen to be produced, not only does the defective cortisol not enable transference storage thyroid (T4) to active thyroid (T3) but the high level total estrogen binds both T3 and T4. As a review, remember, total estrogen should not only include ovarian estrogen, but adrenal estrogens, plant estrogens, called phytoestrogens, and estrogen from plastics, called xenoestrogens.

One day, all health care professionals will realize that elevated estrogen, a lack of thyroid production, and deficient or defective cortisol lead to a loss of bone density, referred to as osteoporosis.

This can occur due to at least three different conditions.

1. The first condition begins with reduced transference from storage thyroid to active thyroid due to the cortisol imbalance.

2. The second condition that occurs is high total estrogen, which further binds both thyroid hormones.

3. The third condition that occurs is due to the high total estrogen that deregulates the immune system, causing an antibody deficiency to occur throughout the mucous membranes of the body, including the gut.

This antibody is called IgA. When the IgA falls below a certain level, oral nutrients, supplements, vitamins, and medications cannot be absorbed properly, including calcium. This is the only deficiency that occurs with the deregulated immune system.

Note: This deregulation of the immune system allows the immune cells (B and T lymphocytes), to lose recognition of self tissue and make antibodies against self tissue, causing autoimmunity and uncontrolled tissue growth.

Between the elevated phosphorus that occurs due to metabolic breakdown, as well as the kidneys' further addition of phosphorus, plus the slowed metabolism and the inability to absorb calcium through the gut, the phosphorus builds up and causes further molecules to be removed from the bones, leading to osteoporosis.

There must be a concern for using an estrogen-containing medication, including birth control pills, because if the total estrogen is not measured before the supplement is given, and if the patient is estrogen prominent, the supplement will cause an estrogen dominance to occur and will push the patient not only into osteoporosis but also into an imbalanced mechanism which could expose the patient to allergies, autoimmunity, and cancer.

It is vital to check males for total adrenal estrogen level so they, too, can be protected from developing osteoporosis, allergies, autoimmunity, and cancer. Remember, all males, whether animals or their owners, have large amounts of estrogen produced from the inner layer adrenal cortex, and when there a cortical imbalance, the pituitary gland will cause the adrenal cortex to producing a damaging amount of adrenal estrogen.

Often, problems with osteoporosis may heighten as a female approaches menopause.

This is due to the fact that she may be given an estrogen supplement based upon the drop in one of the ovarian estrogens, estradiol. But what about adrenal estrogen? It is the amount of total estrogen that needs to be measured, which is a combination of ovarian estrogen and adrenal estrogen, before a patient is put on an estrogen supplement.

If you are still ovulating, to help determine if you are estrogen prominent, have your health care professional take a serum sample on the seventh day of your cycle, when ovarian estrogen is supposed to be at its lowest point of production, and on the twenty-seventh day or whatever day your health care professional recommends, when your ovarian estrogen is the highest. The difference between the two phases of your menstrual cycle will tell you the amount of total estrogen you are producing. Determining these levels may help you avoid developing osteoporosis.

With all the concerns about the damage excess estrogen can cause, no one realizes that the various estrogen measurements during and after ovulation include a large amount of adrenal estrogen.

Many times it is thought the males do not produce estrogen because they have no ovaries! This is **wrong**!

This lack of understanding about adrenal estrogen is why allergies, autoimmunity, and cancer continue on.

The Plechner's Syndrome blood test, the EI1 panel, will give you, your pet, and your health care professionals some very important answers on how to protect you, your family, and your pet from multiple diseases. My question to you is, why not test for this imbalance?

A cortisol replacement is thought to make osteoporosis worse. Do you really think this will occur after you have done the correct tests?

Many health care professionals do not have laboratories that are actually doing total estrogen level testing. So how can you tell where you and your pet might be with this disorder or with almost any chronic disease? You really cannot.

You and your pet definitely do not want to be a statistic based on what some lab tells your health care professional. You are told that you, or your pet, are within the normal empirical range. What does that really mean?

It does not really matter what values are present unless there is a deficiency present. Who really cares how much hormone the lab tells you that you have?

Realize, it does not matter if the hormone levels are normal, because the question is: "Is the hormone active or inactive?" and "Can the hormone in the body actually do its job?"

Even when salivary tests and twenty-four-hour urine tests identify the amounts of free hormone that is present, if the receptor sites are blocked, these free hormones will not be available to the body.

My laboratory studies compare the hormones that regulate the immune system. If the hormones are bound, then this will be reflected by the measurement of specific antibodies.

The day is coming soon, hopefully, when this will be recognized, and you and your pet can regain good health or continue good health once laboratories realize this and begin measuring for these values.

The amount of regulatory hormone therapy will be determined by normalizing the antibody production from the B lymphocyte. The other immune cell, called a T lymphocyte, will also regain function, and both cells will again protect the patient and bring back recognition of self tissue.

A friend of mine has a wife who was so osteoporotic that she could not ride in a car without a special cushion, which helped her to not sustain fractures. After her husband had this endocrine-immune mechanism checked, he found that she not only had the cortisol imbalance, but it was accompanied by a high total estrogen level, bound thyroid hormones, and an IgA deficiency.

Even though most of our health care professionals believe a cortisol supplement is contraindicated, he did do a replacement for her cortisol and a T3 and T4 with hormone supplements. She began to recalcify and could again ride in a car and not sustain pathological fractures.

Until we as healers have answers for treating all diseases, we must keep looking, and because what we find may exist outside the box, or it does not exist because it was not taught in professional school, catastrophic diseases will continue taking life away from innocent people and innocent animals.

Clinical Signs of the Hormonal Antibody Imbalance: Cats

- Simple skin area of inflammation/eosinophilic plaque

- Red, runny eyes part of the year or the entire year

- Chronic inflammation of the ears or hematoma, including yeast, and bacterial infection

- Off and on runny nose

- Sneezing and coughing off and on or all year long

- Chronic vomiting and or diarrhea

- Red gum flare next to the enamel of the tooth

- Personality problems or changes

- Spraying urine in the house even though spayed or neutered

- False pregnancy (this is rare)

- Greasy hair

- Matted hair

- Excess shedding

- Excess licking in general

- Miliary dermatitis

- Neuroma of the bottom lip

- Feline acne of the chin

- Rodent ulcer of the lips

- Allergy

- Autoimmunity

- Cancer

Clinical Signs of the Hormonal Antibody Imbalance: Dogs

There are many subtle effects of this imbalance that are not usually associated with this hormonal antibody imbalance:

- A simple inflammation of an area of skin (hotspot)

- Red runny eyes part of the year or the entire year

- Chronic inflammation of the ears

- Anal gland secretion that occurs and discharges too quickly

- Off and on runny nose

- Sneezing, coughing, and difficult breathing chronically or at certain times of the year

- Vomiting or diarrhea with certain foods (if not highly seasoned or rotten)

- Vomiting or diarrhea with loud noises. (i.e., thunder, fireworks)

- Red gums or bad breath without plaque on the teeth

- Excess pigmentation of the skin of the ventral abdomen and inside the ears

- Thickened and hyper-pigmented areas of skin

- Extreme mood swings including personality problems

- Head shaking—"ear flopping" in the absence of an ear infection or inflammation, especially after barking

- False pregnancy

- Allergies

- Autoimmunity

- Cancer

- Loss of hair in general or loss of patches of hair

- Excess licking in general (i.e., legs, feet, etc.)

- Constipation. To understand this better, one must realize that when cortisol is not working properly and total estrogen is high, not only does this cortisol stop transference from storage thyroid hormone T4 to active thyroid hormone T3, but the high total estrogen binds T3 and T4. Once the thyroid is bound, the peristaltic action in the gut is reduced. This peristalsis of the gut is gut motility. Once the gut motility has slowed, water and toxins are better absorbed because the gut motility is slower. A low-motility gut, being slower with more water reabsorption, turns the stool (excrement) into very hard pieces of material that are hard to pass. Thus, constipation can be the direct result of the hormonal imbalance.

These are just a few of the indications that your dog may have a hormonal antibody imbalance.

Case Studies

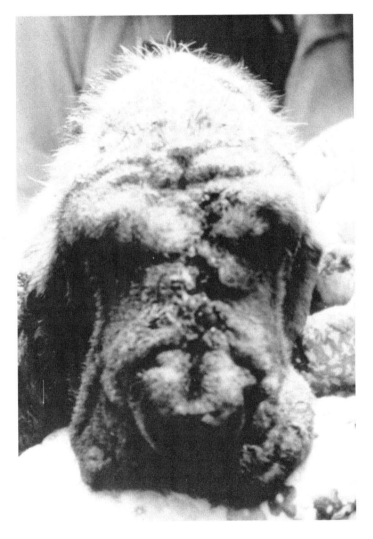

If you ever see a young puppy that looks like this basset hound pup, it probably has Plechner's Syndrome.

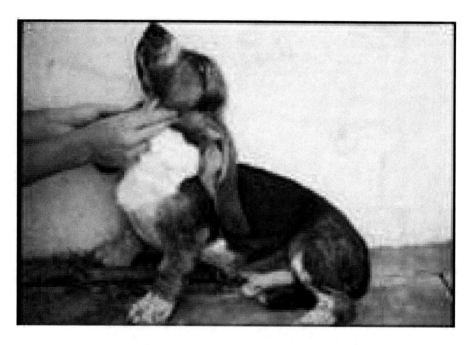

This is the same puppy approximately eight weeks after the start of hormone replace and balancing therapy for his Plechner's Syndrome.

CASE 1

Heidi was a lovely red Doberman Pinscher female belonging to Bill and Marcy Shatner. One weekend, Heidi was admitted to the veterinary hospital with an unsteady gait, dragging her rear legs. The veterinarian on duty quickly decided that this was a case of wobbler syndrome. Wobbler syndrome is an improper amount of supportive ligaments in the neck of the patient. When the patient dropped her head to eat, her cervical vertebrae bodies would put pressure upon her spinal cord due to the ligament instability of the bones of her cervical spine.

The diagnosis was made and euthanasia suggested. I fortunately had worked with the Shatners for a number of years, and they decided to wait out the weekend to discuss this problem Monday morning with me. I had not been contacted over the weekend by the veterinarian for my thoughts and did not know my patient had been hospitalized.

The diagnosis for wobbler syndrome or cervical vertebrae instability should have not been made without sedating the patient and doing a very careful cervical flex of the neck onto chest. Often the flex is not even necessary. A plain lateral X-ray of the neck will often show the cervical instability by actually showing tilted cervical vertebrae bodies. This is usually seen between C4 and C5. Upon examination of Heidi, the gentle flex of the neck caused no pain. She did have a tremendously distended abdomen.

Monday morning Heidi was sent to radiology for me to see why her abdomen was so distended. Upon examination of the X-rays, it was apparent that Heidi was suffering from a horribly upset stomach and intestines. The gas production was monumental. It is interesting in a canine that when abdominal distention is present, the pain from the distention is referred to the rear legs, resulting in a wobbly stance. This is not unlike a heart pain in a human referred down the left arm. Since all the rest of Heidi's vital signs were normal, I worried about a food sensitivity and hormonal antibody imbalance allowing for her food sensitivity. Before actually testing Heidi for hormonal antibody imbalance, I designed a hypoallergenic diet to help Heidi reduce her gastric-intestinal distention.

The food that the Shatners graciously cooked for Heidi was a combination of soybean, brown rice, carrots, and celery. I had Mark Morris, Sr., check out the formulation for long-term use, and Mark suggested using some calcium carbonate. Needless to say, Heidi did return to normal and lived a happy normal life.

Soon thereafter, one Saturday I was seeing patients and I had a similar situation present itself from one of my partners. Fortunately my partner was out of town when the client brought in a beautiful black Doberman male for euthanasia. In reviewing of my partner's X-rays, the prominent pattern was present. I refused to euthanize his pet and asked him to only give one day on this special diet (at that time called the Heidi diet). The patient recovered nicely and proceeded to enjoy normal health and great happiness.

Two years later, I had another patient that responded nicely to the Heidi diet. I was the third veterinarian whom the owner (husband) had visited. He really wasn't quite sure of my recommendations. But after one week he knew this had been the problem the entire time.

Two weeks later, I received a frantic call from the wife telling me her husband was going to the other veterinarian to kill him for the thousand dollars plus he had been charged for **no diagnosis**. I was able to reach the husband on his cell phone and reminded him of the fact that the dog was still alive and viable, and to be thankful. Please amortize the expense over the life of the dog; what he spent for his "best buddy" was cheap at half the price.

CASE 2

Boss was one of the top German Shepherds in the Beverly Hills Police Department's Canine Unit. He was a highly trained canine who had apprehended more than fifty criminals at the time, and twice he won the gold medal for being an outstanding police dog in California. Unfortunately, for the longest time, Boss was of great concern for his handler and best friend, Officer Jay Broyles. I first had the privilege to examine Boss in 1984.

Officer Broyles gave me the following history: Each year in California, the top dogs compete in a Police Dog Olympics. The competition includes obedience tests, obstacle courses, speed drills, and attack skills. Boss won the Olympics in 1982, the first time Office Broyles entered him. This occurred shortly after Boss had been procured from Germany. Unfortunately, within the year that Boss had won this event, he developed lameness in his rear legs that returned from time to time. Unexpectedly during some vigorous activity, he would abruptly stop, pull up lame, and seek the ground in his obvious agony. It would occur after jumping a barrier, during a training session, or while chasing a ball in the backyard. He would suffer for four to six weeks with each episode. This cannot occur on duty where a failure of this magnitude could cost Boss and Officer Broyles their lives.

Officer Broyles related to me that the veterinarian he consulted with had diagnosed Boss's problems as panosteitis (usually a disease that only affects puppies). Panosteitis is a disease of fast-growing canines that may cause a "rotating leg lameness" with radiological evidence of cavitations within the bone itself, and within these cavitations often are allergic white blood cells called eosinophils that point to some kind of an immune response to the puppies' long bones, caused by the puppies' immunes systems being imbalanced

The veterinarian's diagnosis of panosteitis was puzzling because Boss was not a puppy but was three years of age. The veterinarian prescribed a cortisone medication and said Boss would outgrow the condition. Unfortunately Boss did not outgrow the problem.

Office Boyles related the fact that Boss had a couple of incidents like this yearly. Luckily it never happened on the job. He had always performed with great excellence, but he also had a slight inflammation of his skin, and there was always that nagging bit of fear in the back of my mind that something could happen at a critical moment.

The Beverly Hills Police Department obtained Boss when he was two years old. Officer Broyles said, "Boss has worked with me and lived with our family ever since. Once he saved my life by attacking an armed suspect who would otherwise have shot me if Boss hadn't gotten to him. Obviously he is a member of my family. We are very concerned about losing this great animal."

Officer Broyles brought Boss to see me for a third opinion. Unfortunately, if Boss could not do his job in the field, he would be retired and, if in retirement, he suffered too badly with his condition, he should be euthanized.

Officer Broyles told me about the panosteitis diagnosis, which, again, is extremely rare in adult dogs. I was given the opportunity of examining this absolutely elegant dog with such great presence. Upon examination, I did find that Boss had a chronic skin disorder on his back, his abdomen, and his heels. A little known fact is that probably 90 percent of German Shepherds have a digestive enzyme deficiency. I checked Boss's ability to produce the digestive enzyme trypsin. There were no enzymes. This tells me that not only could Boss not absorb calcium, but he also could not absorb other nutrients to guarantee him proper health. The lack of calcium in his bones was now easily explained by his inability to absorb calcium, which would account not only for his panosteitis but also for his dermatitis. His chronic pain and lameness were also part of his enzyme deficiency.

The therapy included diet changes and supplementation with enzymes and calcium. Boss responded dramatically to the program and, in less than two months, Boss appeared to be his "old tough guy" self again. The pain and lameness did not reoccur. Boss's skin problems also cleared up very quickly. His hair coat again retained sheen. He even gained some great muscular weight. Officer Broyles said Boss was more alert now than ever.

Boss improved to such a degree that Officer Broyles decided to enter Boss in the 1985 Police Dog Olympics. Boss had not competed for three years because of his condition. An elated Officer Boyles called me up to report that Boss had beaten out forty-nine other law enforcement dogs and had won the Police Dog Olympics. A few months later, Boss outperformed thirty-two other dogs at the world level and won the World Police & Fire Olympics. Good for Boss!

CASE 3

Over the years I have treated a number of inbred Golden Retrievers who were guide dogs for the blind. Their problems ranged from food sensitivities to severe skin problems and behavioral problems. Unfortunately, it often requires a specialized diet and hormone replacement given orally or by injection to keep this animal in a functional state.

Some of these animals were so seriously genetically defective, there was no way they could handle their responsibilities as guide dogs. What a horrible catastrophe for a sightless person having to stake his or her life on a genetically defective, poor inbred dog that has no hope of fulfilling his or her function.

From my standpoint as a veterinarian and a person who loves spending my life helping animals—and it is very hard not to love all of them—when I find many of these animals have been designed to die no matter what I do, it is tragic!

One such case was a neat Golden Retriever named Edson. Charlene Hunt procured Edson at one and a half years of age. In Charlene's own words, "Edson has been sick for most of the five years that I have had him." This was a dog that was supposed to help maintain Charlene's life and help her substitute her loss of sight, but Edson could not.

Edson developed severe skin sores that many times required treatment twice or three times daily. Can you imagine how hard this was for Charlene to deal with because she could not see him? On a number of occasions, people stopped Charlene in the street accusing her of beating Edson and threatening to call the humane society. At times, the sores were so extreme that Edson could hardly move, and Charlene would have to take a cab home from work with Edson.

Edson also suffered from severe diarrhea when he ate anything but a hypoallergenic diet. Although we were able to stabilize him to some degree, he continued to decline. His inbreeding was such that he had been created to die early in life.

His energy level was never good. Charlene took care of him, but he could not take care of her. This was not his choice.

Unfortunately, at six and a half years of age, Edson had gone from living to existing, with no hope for function, and was put to sleep to stop his suffering. What about Charlene? Edson, unfortunately, was the third dog she had obtained from the same California seeing eye dog facility at that time. Each time the animal, was unable to fulfill his or her functional responsibility for Charlene.

The first dog had behavioral problems, and Charlene had to return the seeing eye dog after three months. The second had hip dysplasia and food sensitivities. Special diets were required. How could Charlene manage this, and why should she have to? This was totally unfair for not only Charlene but also for the poor dogs that she hoped would help her make her way through life being sightless. She again was forced to return another dog because of genetic defects.

"I know of other guide dogs with terrible skin problems and other serious defects," Charlene said. We both informed the school about the existing problems, but the school denied that they had any existing problems. Charlene found that people seemed to be going back to the guide dog school about every two years or so for a new dog. Guide dogs never lasted a good eight to ten years as they should. There is no excuse for this.

Some time ago, I contacted the guide dog school and offered my services at no charge to help them produce healthy, happy dogs for the sight challenged. The guide dog school was not interested.

After Charlene's negative experiences, I suggested she definitely find another guide dog elsewhere. She traveled to an east coast school, hoping for better luck. There, she was assigned a German Shepherd and has had him for over a year without any major problems.

CASE 4

Judy Flerman is a sight-challenged medical secretary who has been a client of mine for years. Note: All treatment costs were modified for the sight challenged, who try so hard and have made a difference. Judy had received a yellow Labrador named Haven. Haven, unfortunately, was sick from the day she arrived. "She was vomiting, practically every day while we were training together at school," Judy recalls. "They told me Haven had a 'nervous' stomach because of all the drilling and classes, but when we got home the vomiting continued two to three times weekly. She was sluggish and would not play."

Unfortunately, Judy had grown much attached to her by then. "For three years, I took her from one veterinarian to another. It was very difficult for me trying to be the eyes of the dog I love and still horribly expensive and still painful to know that Haven was still sick."

"A friend told me about Dr. Plechner, and I took Haven to see him. He was my last resort before giving up! Dr. Plechner tested her hormones and antibodies and recommended a cortisol-thyroid replacement to reestablish her immune system. We started the program, and that was five years ago. She's been healthy ever since. She was kept this way with special foods and replacement hormones. Today, at nine and one-half, she's still able to work. But the day will come when I will have to retire her and find some new 'eyes.' I just dread the prospect and expense of going through this thing again."

I remember the day that Judy's dog froze in the middle of a busy intersection during peak hours, and Judy had to pick up her dog in her arms and wade through traffic with them both at risk of being killed. Can you even imagine what that must have felt like? Good job, Judy! I am very impressed and thankful neither one of them were hurt.

The problems experienced by Charlene Hunt and Judy Flerman are repeated almost daily around the country. They will continue until the schools stop dispensing defective dogs. They provide animals to the blind without cost. But is it really without cost and with no function? Hopefully you will never have to make these decisions.

Whether these guide dog schools breed dogs themselves or accept them as gifts from generous people, these organizations should be concerned about providing healthy animals to those people who are sight-challenged and should not just make money off of the poor people who are handicapped sight-wise.

As Judy Flerman says, "What's the use of all the good intentions if the dogs bring more burden than benefit? The one thing we do not need is more burdens. We should not have to bring sick dogs home, and this is happening frequently enough to make this a very unsettling business."

Clean hips and clean elbows are not enough. These animals need to be clean inside, too. They need certification for normal adrenal cortex function and normal antibody response. The guide dog schools should make every effort to ensure that their animals can serve the handicapped owners without the guide dogs becoming handicapped themselves.

CASE 5

Ardsley was wonderful Cairn Terrier. She was the light of my life and her owner's life. Ardsley had horrible endocrine-immune imbalances. As long as she was maintained on proper hormones plus definite proper diet, she could remain viable.

Any time Ardsley ate a minuscule amount of any food to which her immune cells were reactive, she developed an inflammation of the pancreas. Unfortunately, if this inflammation continues for too long, the pancreas can break down its own ductile system and can release its own enzymes into the gland itself and cause the death of the patient within four to six hours.

Ardsley often would get stomach upsets with no foreign food being supplemented. I worried about stray cats burying their feces in her yard. Many people believe that cats need very high percentages of protein to exist. This is not the case. Much of the protein is passed in the stool because the high level of protein in the food cannot be totally absorbed by the intestines. This is why dogs seek out cat feces—there is undigested food in the feces. This worried me for Ardsley. The owner guaranteed me this was not occurring. Ardsley was very allergic to any products that were not meat. Ardsley was also very allergic to chicken. But no chicken appeared in her non-meat diet. Ardsley's owners were very astute people. One day they discovered that crows and ravens were spending lots of time at the Kentucky Fried Chicken restaurant nearby. As these birds flew across Ardsley's yard, they would occasionally drop a piece of chicken. Ardsley would immediately eat the chicken remains and develop a mysterious pancreatitis.

Everything went very well until, on Halloween evening, Ardsley found the Halloween candy. Unfortunately, because it was a weekend, I was out of town, and poor Ardsley perished. Believe me, it is always hard to lose any patient, especially one you think of as a family member.

78

CASE 6

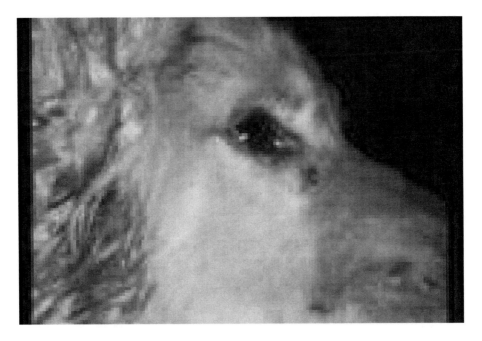

Dune upon commencement of treatment as he first presented to me at my office.

Dune was a wonderful Golden Retriever puppy, ten weeks of age. The poor little guy was probably one of the worst cases of an endocrine-immune balance that I had ever seen. His ears and muzzle were swollen two to three times normal size, bleeding, oozing, and losing hair. He was a very pathetic looking puppy. He tested cortisol deficient, antibody deregulated, plus definitely hypothyroid. He really was the reason I began my search for Plechner's Syndrome.

The breeder of Dune was so upset with his diminished size and other problems that she brought in the mother of Dune, who was a winning show dog. The mother had only experienced an occasional mild dermatitis during the summer. Tests showed that she also had an antibody imbalance. This was her first litter, of only two puppies. Obviously the father had similar imbalances, and when the parents procreated, the imbalances were concentrated in their offspring.

I checked the other puppy, Dune's sibling, and he also had an antibody deficiency. All four dogs had an endocrine-immune imbalance, which included mom, dad, and the two puppies.

Dune probably had other hormone imbalances with growth hormone, etc. He only reached thirty-four pounds even on special diets and hormone regulation of the immune system. I was able to keep my little friend alive for six years. If you had met my little friend, you, too, would have loved his personality and outlook.

This is a case where a parent may be just somewhat off the norm. When the mate is also somewhat abnormal, the genetic flaw seems to magnify and concentrate as this imbalance is passed on to the offspring. Some offspring seem to inherit less while some offspring tend to inherit more. However, both will be affected in some manner. The imbalance can be identified in both parents, and if present, a different breeding is indicated to dilute out the imbalances.

Welcome to Plechner's Syndrome.

Note: You can see actual pictures of Dune on my website under the article button at the second lecture. http://drplechner.com/pdf/plechner-lecture-02.pps I took these slides of Dune in 1971, and my studies are only just now being considered, almost forty years later.

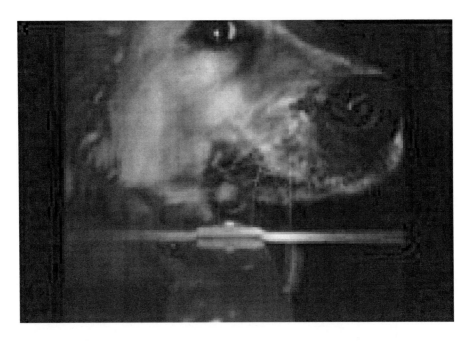

Dune after approximately two weeks of hormonal rebalancing treatment.

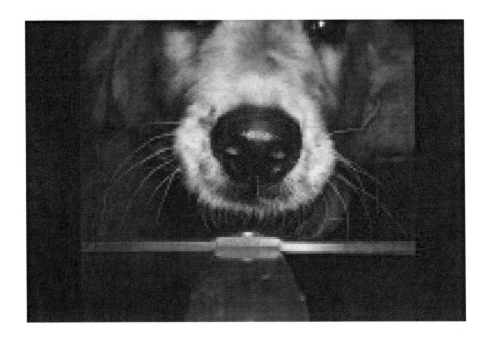

CASE 7

Tuesday was an eight-year-old spayed female feline. She was a grey and orange domestic short hair. At eight years of age, she had surgery for a malignant mammary tumor (carcinoma). At this point in her life, the owner was told that Tuesday had only two weeks to live. The owner had heard about my endocrine-immune studies and scheduled an office call. Upon examination, the cat purred and wanted to be fondled. She was an elegant cat that just wanted to live.

In reviewing the history with the owner, no tumor spread had been discovered or identified at the time of surgery. The area of surgery was slightly bumpy, but nothing was found out of the ordinary. I did an EI1 panel (Plechner's Syndrome) and found that Tuesday was classic for the mechanism defect for all cancer patients. Her cortisol was defective, her total estrogen was high, her thyroid hormones were bound, and her immune cells were deregulated. Normally a cat only needs a cortisol replacement to normalize the hormones and re-regulate her immune system.

After two weeks, the endocrine-immune imbalance began to correct itself. During this time no tumor growth appeared at the surgery site. After four weeks of hormone replacement, the endocrine-immune mechanism returned to normal.

In six years of the therapy, Tuesday was normal with no more cancer.

At fifteen years of age, Tuesday began to develop diabetes mellitus. As a patient ages, his or her normal hormone production, along with the replacement hormone, may lessen in its production, and an increase in endogenous hormone may be indicated. If this is the situation, then many times a lack of hormone increase may allow the slightly deregulated immune cells to lose recognition of self breakdown products but also can make anti-antibody to various hormones including insulin.

Many in my profession believe that cortisol, even if deficient in a patient, causes an insulin deficiency. This is definitely wrong and has been proven to be wrong.

I did refer Tuesday to a specialist to handle this secondary diabetes. The first thing the veterinary specialist said to the owner was, "You must stop the cortisol." This is often done, and the patient usually dies because he or she needs the replacement hormone to live, including their deficiency in insulin. I was able to convince the specialist to adjust the insulin levels for Tuesday and continue my therapy, and now Tuesday is eighteen years old and doing very well. Hormone levels are checked every six months and appear to be normal with no signs of recurrent cancer.

CASE 8

Archie is a bright orange tomcat, probably one year old, with bright yellow eyes and a great fondness for all people. He is the kind of cat you must watch carefully so you do not trip over him as he is rubbing up against you.

Unfortunately, Archie was exposed to the feline leukemia virus, and he had Plechner's Syndrome, which allowed for him to develop feline leukemia. Cats that do not have Plechner's Syndrome, which is an endocrine-immune imbalance, will not develop any of the retroviruses like feline leukemia, feline immunodeficiency virus, or feline infectious peritonitis.

Those cats with a partial imbalance, if exposed to any of these retroviruses, may become positive for the virus and may even shed the virus but will not develop the actual disease. Once the endocrine-immune imbalance is identified and funded, 85 percent of all cats that have feline leukemia can live a normal life and attain a normal life span.

Archie was treated for his leukemia with only a cortisol replacement. He did very well. Fortunately, he was in the 85 percent. Three months of replacement cortisol and reregulation of his immune cells protected him against the leukemia virus and allowed him to reach maturity.

Archie lived to be twenty-eight years of age. He was a happy, very gracious cat. His only hang-up was that he enjoyed roaming the neighborhood picking up stray kittens. I must have placed over twelve kittens that Archie carried home over that twenty-eight-year period.

What a great experience for me to have known and helped Archie!

CASE 9

Kiddo was a two-year-old breeding Abyssinian cat with striking features of his golden orange coat. Kiddo's problem was that he continually produced bladder stones (gravel) that would block him from passing urine normally.

Upon doing an endocrine-immune panel, I found Kiddo had the imbalance that allowed for stone production. Kiddo was pretty typical of cats with this imbalance. His cortisols were imbalanced, his total estrogen elevated, his T3 and T4 (thyroid hormones) were bound, and his immune cells were deregulated. All his antibody production was deficient, including the IgA level, which, when normal, protects all the mucous membranes in the body. Kiddo's IgA mucous membrane antibodies were nonexistent. Therefore, the bladder not being protected by nonexistent IgA also opens the gut mucous membrane to the same danger. With the bowel being challenged, absorption is also challenged. It appears carbohydrate is more easily absorbed then protein. Remember, carbohydrate creates alkaline urine, and protein creates acidic urine. Kiddo's mucous membrane (IgA) antibody is nonexistent; therefore, the urine is alkaline.

In alkaline urine, soluble minerals (minerals in solution) precipitate into the urine. With imbalanced cortisol, the elevated estrogen causes inflammation of most linings of arteries (endothelia cells) in the body. Therefore, cells in the medulla of kidneys, called juxtaglomerular cells, produce excess mucous that binds the bladder stones and causes a toothpaste-like tubular wedge of material that will occlude the smallest exit opening from the bladder.

Unfortunately, the male cat normally has the smallest diameter urethra going through the penis from the bladder. Female cats normally have a short, wide urethra leading from the bladder to outside the body. Many in my profession believe that if you remove the penis in a male cat and enlarge the diameter of the urethra, this mucous-stone paste will pass out and not obstruct the patient, which is true; however, the IgA imbalance will still exist without hopefully causing further urinary obstruction. The condition still exists. The medical effect has been helped with surgery, but the cause has not. I was able to help Kiddo without removing his penis (called post-pubic urethrostomy). The problem with so many animals is that they have Plechner's Syndrome and, when bred, they pass the imbalance to their offspring.

Just recently, it is now believed that idiopathic lower urinary syndrome comes from an adrenal imbalance. My profession may be slowly learning. I certainly hope so for the health of the animals.

CASE 10

I remember examining a Burmese Mountain dog that was probably the number one show dog in America. He had sired 270 puppies all over the US.

Upon examination for Buddy's rear leg lameness, I found that he had very severe hip dysplasia, which is usually a genetic defect.

Hip dysplasia, for your information, is the genetic hip and femoral head malformation that may not show any of these radiological changes on X-ray until after two years of age. The condition leads to a shallow or nonexistent hip socket with an irregular femoral head and a very short, crooked femoral neck. All degrees of hip dysplasia can occur, from a very slight structural change to a total subluxation of both femoral heads.

I first discovered a form of hip dysplasia in 1967 when I had a chance to check X-rays of many German dogs. At this time the Germans did not think they had a problem. Instead of relating to the X-rays of their dogs and the mild structural changes in the bones that were evident, they would run their dogs ten miles while on bicycles. If the dog did not show any signs of lameness, then the Germans considered the dog normal and a definite candidate to breed.

One problem with hip dysplasia is that the parent can have horrible hips and no signs of the disease, including pain. However, in the offspring, the disorder can be catastrophic. Even with parents that have been officially cleared, the gene for the problem can exist in the parents without skeletal signs and can definitely manifest this gene in the offspring.

CASE 11

A breeder had contacted me, concerned that her three-year-old breeding pair of Vizslas (canines), or Hungarian Pointers, had developed a terminal cancer (malignancy) of the spleen referred to a hemangiosarcoma. Hemangiosarcomas are extremely malignant tumors that develop in the endothelium, the lining of the blood vessels, and the spleen. Death usually occurs within a few months of life as a result of metastasis (spread of the tumor) to the right atrium of the heart. Ultrasound determined that no metastasis had occurred. In each case of a splenic mass, usually surgery and excision is performed.

I tested both dogs for an endocrine-immune imbalance (Plechner's Syndrome) and found that both were imbalanced, as all cancer patients are, whether animal or human. The male was badly imbalanced, with a mucous membrane antibody (IgA) so low that malabsorption would occur. An injection of hormone was indicated to bypass the gut. The female was also imbalanced in the same endocrine-immune areas.

Proper medication and administration of the hormones were indicated, and within one month the imbalances in both dogs had been normalized. Both dogs were field trial champions before this occurred. Both dogs have been maintained on this hormonal rebalance program since that time and are in good health and happily involved in hunting again.

Remember, when both parents are affected by this imbalance, the imbalance will be concentrated in their offspring. This is why it is so important to check for Plechner's Syndrome with both parents. If they are both imbalanced in the same area, that imbalance will be concentrated in the offspring. Therefore, look for a different breeding mate. If both parents are imbalanced in different endocrine-immune areas, the defects may be lessened in their offspring. The lesson to learn here is, because one or both parents test positively for Plechner's Syndrome, it is not to say don't breed these dogs, just do not breed these dogs together. Find different mates!

When parents have similar imbalances, as these dogs did, experience has shown that the offspring will likely have the same abnormalities and are at high risk of developing the same cancer.

The male and female Vizslas had produced a litter of six puppies about one year before their operations for hemangiosarcoma.

Shortly after treating the parents of these one-year-old puppies, four males and two females, the puppies were tested for Plechner's Syndrome. Remember, if you test the cause before these bad effects occur, the correction of the EI imbalance will result in stopping an eventual medical effect that can range from allergies to autoimmunity and cancer. The puppies each had the same endocrine-immune imbalance that allowed for cancer to develop in their parents.

The breeder agreed that the best preventative strategy was to normalize these imbalances with a proper hormone replacement program. The young dogs were placed on a combination of cortisol and thyroid based upon their weight. The last report I received was that the parents were thirteen years old and the puppies eight years old, and all were doing fine.

For a much more in-depth look at this study, please go to my compendium of articles on my website, page 39. The article is entitled, "Innovative Cancer Therapy That Saves Animals, May Protect Humans As Well."

CASE 12

Bob was an eight-year-old, male, neutered Siberian husky. In June of 2003, I had the privilege of treating Bob. Two months earlier, a previous veterinarian had diagnosed Bob with multiple metastatic lung tumors (Bob had multiple growths in his lungs), but the site of this primary cancer had not been identified so far. The veterinarian expected Bob to die as all the others have done with this same kind of cancer. Bob was eating poorly, breathing with difficulty, and coughing persistently. Bob had lost twelve pounds of weight since the original diagnosis.

I suggested doing an endocrine-immune test and the owner asked me to medicate Bob even before the test results came back. As I mentioned, all cancer patients have an easily identified endocrine imbalance (Plechner's Syndrome) that can be corrected to control the cause of the cancer. This is definitely not to say the effects of cancer should not be treated, but this combination including identifying and controlling the cause of why the cancer has occurred, allows all the patients a better chance to survive, whether they are animals or humans.

Bob began his hormone-immune rebalance control treatment. Two weeks later, the owner returned with a healing Bob. He had regained four pounds and was breathing easier. I rechecked his blood levels. The key elevated estrogen and deficient antibodies levels had improved significantly. In two more weeks, I had rechecked his blood levels, and they were even closer to normal. Thoracic X-rays revealed that the lung lesion had disappeared. There was no visual evidence of lung tumors. Bob now weighed his normal seventy-eight pounds, and not only regained his appetite but was also able to breathe normally.

Although Bob has been on therapy for only a short period of time, the initial response has been excellent and not unusual. The potential exists for normal health for Bob as long as he maintains the treatment program. I did suggest rechecking blood levels every three months and then yearly.

The best treatment of any disease lies in its prevention. Bob was lucky.

Without identifying Plechner's Syndrome first, often the radiation can further damage the body's hormone production while deregulating an already dysfunctional immune system. Now you have both endocrine and immune systems damaged and survival will be very questionable.

CASE 13

Nelly, a female three-year-old spayed Old English Sheepdog, was presented to me with a severe localized inflammation, or swelling of the skin over the spine. It appeared to be a black widow bite. If there had been more tissue destruction, the bite might have come from a brown recluse spider. A therapy program of antibiotics, anti-inflammatory, plus topical Montmorillonite (special clay) proved successful.

However, a month after the black widow bites, Nelly began to lose hair and break out in welts. Nelly then developed diarrhea and vomiting after eating her normal food. An endocrine-immune panel identified the fact that the black widow toxin had damaged the middle layers of the adrenal cortex and its production of normal cortisol.

Soon it will be understood by the general public and health care professionals that most toxins, anesthetics, vaccines, alcohol, heavy metals, radiation, etc. can lead to this suppression or damage to the middle layer adrenal cortex, reduce the production of normal cortisol, and cause the patient to develop Plechner's Syndrome.

Interestingly enough, Nelly's endocrine-immune status had been tested a year earlier and was perfectly normal. Apparently, as already stated, the black widow toxin temporarily compromised the cortisol synthesis pathway enough to cause the hormonal antibody imbalance. Once Nelly began replacement hormone therapy, the clinical signs quickly resolved. A subsequent EI1 test yielded improved values. The combination of active exogenous and endogenous glucocorticoids brought the immune markers back to a level that reestablished immune competence.

At the present time, Nelly has been maintained on the same corrective program for four years and has experienced no health problems. Periodic EI1 testing has revealed normal immune valves. This is a good example of how a toxin can create some level of permanent damage to the middle layer adrenal cortex.

This is not a case caused by genetic damage to the middle layer adrenal cortex. This case points to an external agent that has caused the damage and interrupted the function of the middle layer adrenal cortex; this can be a temporary suspension. The middle layer adrenal cortex may return to near-normal function, and no long-term replacement hormone therapy is indicated in such cases. Doing the EI1 test (Plechner's Syndrome) over time will confirm this.

CASE 14

Miles was a wonderful, very large Airedale Terrier that lived with Kirk Nims, or should I say that Kirk lived with Miles. NOTE: All of my patients are considered to be members of the family. Otherwise I will not get involved.

Miles had all the attributes of a great Airedale but unfortunately had an aggression problem even toward his owners. Kirk joined a rescue parade each year, and Miles could be quite aggressive. At one hundred pounds, this was dangerous. Miles was a very large Airedale by any standard.

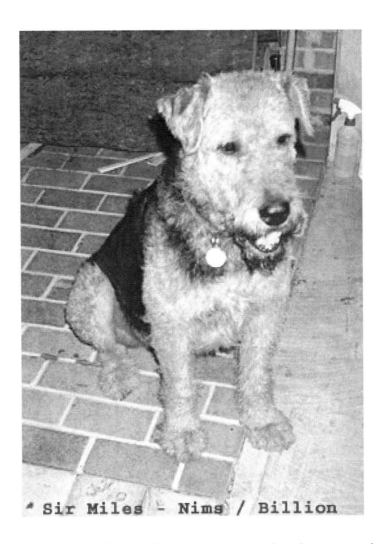

Sir Miles - Nims / Billion

I am not sure exactly how Kirk got to me, but after doing an endocrine-immune panel on Miles, I found that Miles' high estrogen was the reason for the aggression. Once medicated and fed the proper diet, Miles became the Airedale that he wanted to be and should have been.

Kirk also realized there were many Airedales with problems that need not impair their lives. Kirk and Sidney Hardie put together a data collection system on

Airedales and developed a Yahoo! groups website for Airedale Terrier Endocrine Immune Testing: http://pets.groups.yahoo.com/group/ADTEIT/.

The excitement for me was not only being of value to Miles but appreciating the care that the Airedale rescue humans have for the Airedale members of their families. I had not realized when I got involved with Kirk Nims and Debbie Carley with their super Airedale terriers that I was beginning to work with one of the most caring groups of all, the Airedale rescue people, around the world.

After I had hopefully helped the beautiful family member of Kirk Nims and Debbie Carley, they had recommended me to Sue and Bill Forrester and their three Airedales, Alice, Ascha, and Aemon, who lived in Australia. I never did have the opportunity to meet Aemon face to face, but had great pictures of him and also a wonderful love for him. I was given the privilege to help Aemon even after all other therapies failed.

I was practicing at the time in southern California and corresponding with Sue and her veterinarian in Australia. Aemon had a self-immune disorder, referred to as autoimmune hemolytic anemia, that allowed his immune cells to lose recognition of self tissue and self breakdown tissue. He had developed Plechner's Syndrome.

As these deregulated immune cells removed the majority of Aemon's red blood cells from his general circulation, Aemon became close to death. With the help of Sue, Bill, Aemon, and their veterinarian, we tested Aemon and found that he did have low cortisol leading to high total estrogen, which bound his thyroid hormones. The high total estrogen caused deregulation of Aemon's immune cells, which led to their lack of recognition of his red blood cells, which in turn allowed this deregulation to remove his red blood cells and treat this self material as a foreign substance.

As part of the immune deregulation, antibody production from the B lymphocyte becomes deficient. If the antibody deficiency is below a certain level in the gastrointestinal tract (IgA), malabsorption of oral replace hormones occurs.

Also, this deficient level of IgA allows the body to overreact to foods, vaccines, and stinging insect bites.

When Aemon was in the hospital on intravenous fluids and hormones, his red blood cell count increased. Aemon's general health improved dramatically. The main reason for the success was that in the intravenous fluid there were large amounts of soluble cortisol, the lack of which caused Plechner's Syndrome and the domino effect that occurred.

After Aemon returned home, he was placed on a hypoallergenic diet and given oral hormone supplements. Unfortunately, due to the low antibody production in his gut, he malabsorbed not only the food but the oral replacement hormones as well, causing him to get sick again because the nutrients and drugs were not passing through the gut wall. Obviously, Aemon's condition deteriorated in a big hurry.

After several intramuscular injections of a long-acting cortisol, Aemon's endocrine-immune system returned to normal, thus allowing oral hormone supplementation to be effective. Aemon's gut could now absorb. Once the intramuscular cortisols reduced the pituitary impact on the inner layer adrenal cortex, the estrogen level dropped. The high estrogen level was the original reason there was a suppression of all the antibodies including the IgA.

NOTE: Low IgA is the prime reason that patients can be hospitalized and given intravenous or intramuscular injection of necessary antibiotics or any medication. However, when they go home on oral medication, their health problems return because their IgA levels are never checked. Hopefully the day will come when, with every regular blood sample taken, an IgA level will be done also to make sure that what is prescribed for the patient can be absorbed orally.

A plant-based digestive enzyme was suggested for Aemon to make sure his hypoallergenic diet would be properly broken down and allow for maximum absorption for all the nutrients in his food. Please realize that if Aemon's food was not broken down completely, and a sludging effect occurred, his gut would be coated with non-broken-down foods that would stop absorption of his primary hormones, reducing their effectiveness. If this occurred, Aemon's autoimmunity would return.

It is a known fact that improper amounts of cortisol, when leading to its deficiency, will not transfer a bound, storage thyroid to an active thyroid, which the body must have. Therefore, a state of hypothyroid begins to exist. It is further known that high total estrogen will cause actual binding of active thyroid, further complicating the disorder.

What normally is not recognized, when treating a person or animal with long-term replacement cortisol, is that you must use a thyroid compound to guarantee that the daily cortisol replacement is totally broken down in twenty-four hours so that at the time of the administration of the next daily dose, there is no cortisol left from the day before.

You can now understand why in people and animals without thyroid therapy, a buildup of cortisol or other replacement hormones will occur. This is why cortisol, even though it is a natural adrenal cortex hormone, has gotten a bad reputation. It is mainly because the professionals do not realize that if they are not funding thyroid hormone, cortisol therapy will lead to an overdose while giving a cortisol replacement long-term.

One then wonders if the use of Premarin in women allowed for its buildup and catastrophic effects due to a lack of thyroid hormone replacement, so that instead of funding a daily estrogen imbalance, there was Premarin retention in twenty-four hours and, after a number of days, the increased amounts caused catastrophic diseases to occur in those patients taking the drug.

CASE 15

I was given the opportunity to treat a lovely three-year-old spayed female Golden Retriever. She had suffered from puppyhood and through young adulthood with varying degrees of pustular dermatitis. Upon testing her for Plechner's

Syndrome, she did present with low cortisol, high total estrogen, bound thyroid hormones, and a deregulated immune system.

The immune system is thought to be made up of two major components. The B cell, when regulated correctly, protects the body against bacterial infections and makes proper antibodies to vaccines and other foreign invaders. The other major component of the immune system is the T cell. This immune cell, when properly regulated, protects the body against viruses and fungi, i.e., *Candida*. When deregulated, the protection from these agents is damaged. When the B and T cells are deregulated, as you remember, they can turn against the body and make unprotected systems even worse.

Upon analysis of the test results, oral medications were indicated for the Golden Retriever. The deregulation of the B cell was not so severe as to alter the mucous membrane antibody in the gut to disallow for absorption. Intramuscular injections were not necessary. The canine patient responded nicely. Unfortunately, three months later, the owner's brother-in-law, who was a health care professional, persuaded the owner into believing that I was killing his dog. The facts of the case were explained to the owner's brother in law to no avail. The replacement hormones were stopped.

One year later, I received a telephone call from Dr. Gary Rachelefsky, who had been head of Pediatric Allergies at UCLA and was now in private practice. Dr. Rachelefsky had seen a client of mine a few years earlier who owned a canine with a hormonal antibody imbalance.

Dr. Rachelefsky had examined a young girl with a serious bacterial infection on her face called impetigo. Several other pediatricians had identified the bacterial infection as staphylococcus aureus but thought probably the child had an immune deregulation. No other source was identified. Dr. Rachelefsky asked me if I thought the source of the child's infection could come from her dog, a spayed female Golden Retriever. I did agree that the dog certainly could be the source of the infection. I decided to do a bacterial culture from the dog to see if the dog was the source.

The owner of the dog made an appointment to see me. Interestingly enough, this was the canine patient I had worked up and treated before, the one whose owner's brother-in-law said I was killing with my hormone replacement. The bacterial culture I did on the canine turned out to be the same bacteria that Dr. Rachelefsky found on the child.

Young children can be very susceptible to staph infection from dogs and cats. Needless to say, the canine was placed back on the same replacement hormones in order to reregulate the immune cells to protect the canine against uncontrolled bacterial growth. Within two weeks, now that the source had been treated, both patients moved on with their lives.

This case was one of the reasons that caused me to retire, out of pure frustration, and move to the mountains of Idaho.

I have identified a simple blood test that identifies the cause of many catastrophic diseases ranging from allergies to autoimmune to cancer in animals and people. All cancer patients tested have Plechner's Syndrome, whether canine, feline, equine, or human.

What many health care specialists generally do not believe is that the endocrine system, in fact, regulates the immune system.

Since total estrogen serum levels have been such of great concern for the health care specialists, why then are the laboratories only measuring partial estrogens in people and animals? In females, three and only three ovarian estrogens are measured with no realization that a huge amount of adrenal estrogen can be produced from the inner layer adrenal cortex when an imbalance is present. In males, only one partial estrogen is usually measured. They need to consider all the other estrogen that is either produced from the inner layer of the adrenal cortex, ingested from plants (phytoestrogens), and that comes from plastics (xenoestrogens).

Certain food sources contain a partial estrogen called estradiole. This is contained in most foods made from soybeans. You can imagine if you are estrogen dominant and then eat soybean products, it could put you into estrogen dominance and Plechner's Syndrome.

Hopefully you can understand why total estrogen is so very important.

Often the ratio of ovarian estrogens when measured will indicate that one of these estrogens is diminished in quantity; therefore, the patient is given an estrogen supplement. The patient may be high in total estrogen and the replacement estrogen can lead to a catastrophe. Often females also produce elevated male hormone from their inner layer adrenal cortex, called androgen. This often is the reason some women have facial hair. This may be unsightly and have to be dealt with cosmetically, but the real problem may lie with an enzyme that resides in the fatty tissue of a recipient! It just happens that in fatty tissue, an enzyme exists called aromatase that can change androgen into estrogen, which can further disrupt health. It appears that since aromatase occurs in fatty tissue, the heavier the patient is, the greater amounts of aromatase may exist. Again, this may allow for a greater amount of total estrogen to be created, leading to major disease.

The incidence of cancer appears to be rising in people and animals. Is it because diagnostic skills are becoming more efficient, or is it in part due to plastic water pipes and plastic bottled drinks producing more xenoestrogens, or just from environmental exposure to pesticides that mimic the effects of excess estrogen?

CASE 16

Dirk was a neutered male mixed canine, a great dog with a great family. The head of the household was a retired Army colonel with a great sense of humor and personality. He would bring Dirk into my practice for periodic stories and to show off his various implements. The colonel's last appearance was to show me his belt buckle, which was a 22-caliber Derringer gun. I never knew what the colonel would come up with next.

As it turned out, Dirk had food sensitivities and skin allergies due to a hormonal antibody imbalance. Once controlled, his skin problem disappeared, but his sensitivity to certain foods still remained as they usually do. Often it is thought that if you purge your system from a food you are sensitivity to for three to four weeks, thereafter you can eat small amounts of that offending food and you will tolerate that food. However, my experiences have shown me that my patients, after purging their system from a specific offending food, when again eating that food receive an even a worse reaction than they did when that food caused their initial reaction.

Interesting enough, when Dirk tried a new food that he had not been exposed to, the only reaction that occurred was a small amount of occult blood (blood in urine found only through testing) appeared in his urine. So any time a new food was introduced to Dirk, the son would bring in a urine sample for analysis for occult blood.

Food sensitivities come from Plechner's Syndrome and deficient IgA. Since this is the case, in whatever part of the body is not protected by this mucous membrane antibody, a reaction may occur. Dirk's impact area was related to the kidneys where the IgA was deficient and allowed for past sensitivities to occur.

Classically, the skin reaction that occurs due to a food sensitivity usually effects the ears, eyes, feet, and skin on the abdomen. The reason the reaction occurs in these specific areas is because these are the areas where mast cells, which contain histamine, are concentrated. Once the mass cells release their histamine, the inflammation is caused, thus inflammation occurs in those specific areas. If the reaction is more severe in one ear or one paw, it usually means there are more mast cells distributed there.

It is important to realize in animals and people that a food can cause a delayed reaction of up to seven days. If no reaction occurs during the first six days, do not be fooled, because the reaction may occur on the seventh day.

Often, in the history from the owner, I find the patient's reaction occurred a week later. The owner claims he or she did not introduce any new foods, "but last week I did give one cracker." Obviously the reaction did not occur that day or soon after but did occur a week later.

I would then check Dirk's urine on the eighth day to determine if he reacted to the food. If Dirk's occult blood in his urine had not been diagnosed and monitored, his kidney bladder disease might have been catastrophic.

It is thought there are in an animal one million functional kidney units, called nephrons, in each kidney. After months or years of inflammation due to a food sensitivity and hormonal imbalance, these nephrons can be replaced with scar tissue. After there is enough scarring of the kidneys, for these organs to filter out nitrogenous waste products, more urine must be produced to get the job done, and that is when you realize your pet has increased water consumption.

It relates to more blood filtration occurring through fewer nephrons. As time and the damage continue, the dog or cat will have to drink much more fluid. Often protein and glucose may follow with significant weight loss if there is physical or disease processes affecting the kidneys. This occurs most frequently in felines. It often is referred to as chronic interstitial nephritis.

When Plechner's Syndrome causes significant reduction of the protective antibody IgA, anywhere this antibody is reduced, major disease can occur. The reduction in this antibody occurs in all mucous membranes in the body including the digestive tract, respiratory tract, urinary tract, and genital tract. Any surface or organ covered with or contained with this mucous membrane and its antibody can develop diseases with this antibody deficiency. When the imbalance occurs, often the site of the disease is genetically predetermined. This is one reason we may see family traits for developing allergies, autoimmunity, and cancer in specific areas.

All these people and animals have the predisposition for developing the effects of this predictable and preventable hormone imbalance called Plechner's Syndrome. Obviously, identifying the imbalance before the imbalance allows for a disease is the challenge. I have done many animal studies on the offspring of diseased parents, and with funding the hormonal antibody imbalance and avoiding the disease of the parents totally or at least delaying its onset until so late in life, the problem is not a factor. Many times, both prospective parents, upon testing, may have only a slight imbalance. However, if these imbalances are both in the same area, the subclinical imbalance often is transferred to offspring, which causes eventual clinical disease. In animals, it is easy to help the breeder use different parents to avoid problems in the offspring.

In people it does not work this way, but what would be of value would be to test the prospective parents, which might indicate what health issue might accompany their offspring. Once the maternal antibody has left the child, Plechner's Syndrome could be tested for, and if there is an imbalance, it could be corrected before a medical effect develops. Hopefully the day will come when this hormone antibody test will be used as a health check from birth to death in animals and people.

Anytime blood tests, twenty-four-hour urine tests, or salivary tests are done, the endocrine-immune panel (Plechner's Syndrome) should be done to determine if the free hormones can even be used by the body.

CASE 17

Another family had had a beloved male canine that died at eighteen months of age from a vaccine-preventable disease, called parvovirus. He had been vaccinated correctly and repeated the vaccine a number of times. The pet died anyway. You ask yourself, how can that happen? If proper immunization is done in people and animals, the only way of making sure that the patient has made protective antibodies is to the measure antibody levels. This is not routinely done.

The same family decided to adopt a dog from a rescue organization. Gwenovere was a black and white Great Dane puppy referred to as a Harlequin Great Dane. I had the pleasure of checking the puppy to make sure was sound. She was a ten-week-old female with an outgoing personality. Her health appeared to be normal; however, the owners wanted a guarantee that the puppy would not succumb to parvovirus. I vaccinated the puppy myself and gave the owners a list of restrictions to follow. The main restriction was not to expose her to areas that strange dogs frequent, like dog parks. It is okay to expose your new puppy to friends and relatives' dogs that you know have had good health hygiene and have been properly vaccinated.

Two weeks after Gwenovere had her last injection for parvovirus, distemper, etc., I checked her antibody levels. They were nonexistent. These situations are often thought to be caused by a damaged vaccine. This usually is not the cause. As you remember, when there is an endocrine-immune imbalance, antibody production is suppressed. Obviously, a vaccine program will be unproductive antibody-wise if this imbalance exists. I tested the puppy for Plechner's Syndrome and found that the hormonal imbalance was present. Gwenovere was placed on proper hormone replacement and revaccinated. Now that her immune system had returned to normal, the vaccine then did allow the immune system to produce proper protective antibodies. Her titers for parvovirus and distemper had reached proper titer levels for protection of the puppy.

Gwenovere is normal now and will continue to remain so, as long as her hormone replacement is increased as needed as she grows and ages.

Many of our feline patients suffer from the same imbalances that we see with our canine patients. Because of their imbalances and because of the tremendous number of viruses that exist in the feline world, cats are famous for developing some very catastrophic diseases, even after being properly vaccinated. Again, with vaccinations, it now is easily understood why many cats cannot make protective antibodies to diseases for which vaccinations are commonly available.

There is a group of particularly fatal viruses in cats, called retroviruses. This group contains the feline leukemia virus, the feline infectious peritonitis virus, and the feline AIDS virus. Often the retroviruses have associated vaccines available for use, but when the cat is vaccinated, due to the endocrine-immune imbalance, no protective antibodies can be produced. And the animal can develop a retrovirus if exposed.

It is very important to note that a patient can test positive for Plechner's Syndrome, but if the imbalance is only slight, the disease might never develop. However, the cat can still remain as a carrier. If there ever is a question that your cat might have the imbalance and has been exposed, and tests positive, do the EI1 Plechner's Syndrome blood test and correct the imbalance before the disease develops.

This may explain why a person who is HIV-positive may never develop AIDS, if his or her hormonal imbalance is not too severe.

CASE 18

This is an example of a cat that had developed feline leukemia at six months of age. His name was Bob. Bob had lost a lot of weight due to diarrhea, causing a total weakness. His lymph nodes were normal at this time.

When diagnosed with any of the three viruses mentioned in Case 17, even though they are thought to be totally fatal and euthanasia often is thought to be the treatment of choice, this is not true!

After testing, it was quite evident that Bob had the imbalance and, as I mentioned before, with this deregulated immune system, the T cell will not protect his body against any virus. The same conditions exist with feline AIDS and feline infectious peritonitis.

Often, since all antibody production is reduced, including IgA, oral medications are usually malabsorbed. Intravenous and intramuscular injections are indicated with any catastrophic disease even before test levels return, because you cannot assume oral medication will reach the bloodstream through the gut. Injections of the cortisol replacement were given in the muscle at a ten-day interval until the immune system responded and the elevated the IgA antibody allowed for absorption of the oral hormone replacement. Soon Bob's endocrine-immune imbalance returned to normal status and was continued with oral hormone replacements.

Now that the function of the T lymphocyte returned to normal and protected Bob, his blood test became negative for the leukemia virus. He is still living a normal life at fifteen years of age and will as long as he continues to test at the proper hormone levels identified by regular EI1 tests.

CASE 19

As I have already mentioned, I treated a similar large, orange tomcat that began oral therapy at eight months of age. Archie did very well. As a matter of fact, Archie did too well.

Archie would roam the neighborhood and pick up stray kittens and bring them home. You can guess who had to find homes for these kittens. Archie lived twenty-eight years on cortisol replacement.

Cats usually take only cortisol in 90 percent of the cases. Dogs usually take a cortisol replacement with T4 only. People usually take a cortisol replacement with T3 and T4. Horses usually only take T4.

These species variations reflect the different needs of different species, necessitating the use of different hormonal supplements to recreate a healthy endocrine immune system that is in balance.

In cats with retrovirus, the following results can generally be expected: FELV = 85 percent success rate. FIV = 70 percent success rate. FIP = 70 percent success rate, but beside the usual cortisol replacement will also need T4 (thyroid) supplement twice daily.

The clinical pictures may vary slightly with these three viruses, but in some ways they are quite similar.

FIP can produce a wet form or a dry form. With the wet form, there usually is a major production of a straw-like fluid in the abdominal cavity and or in the thoracic cavity. The dry form of FIP does not cause this fluid production. The wet form of FIP is usually noticed more quickly by the owner due to the distention caused by the fluid in the abdomen or the fluid causing compression of the lungs, which leads to noticeable labored breathing.

Remember, if any of these patients are checked for exposure to any of these three retroviruses, they may not have the ability to produce measurable antibody production against any of these viruses, but they can still have the disease. With these cats, even with a history of prior vaccinations, they usually have no protective effect for them due to the imbalance and a depressed antibody production.

The next question that arises is what to do with a cat that is positive for any of these retroviruses? Is he or she a carrier, and can this be contagious to other cats? These viruses are usually only contagious to cats with Plechner's Syndrome.

This is probably why a cat with a normal endocrine-immune system will not develop the disease. This is probably why vaccines for these viruses are of very little value to a normal cat. The vaccines, however, stimulate proper immunity in these cats and may help reduce the viral population.

What to do with a cat that is positive for one of these three viruses?

Short-term isolation, if possible, is indicated unless the positive cat has lived with his other family cats for awhile. Each cat in the household needs to be checked for the three viruses. If the other cats are negative for the virus, they should be watched carefully and possibly vaccinated.

If any of the cats test positive for any of the retroviruses, then an endocrine-immune panel EI1 serum test needs to be done. If the tests are normal, merely watch the cat or cats for any clinical changes, i.e., appetite, loose stools, weight loss, etc.

If any of the cats are positive for a retrovirus, then hormone replacement needs to be started immediately and usually continued thereafter. Often the cat or cats will shed the virus and test negative for any of these viruses after the endocrine-immune homeostasis has returned to normal.

If the cat is identified as positive and no replacement therapy is done, and the cat lives a normal life, then the endocrine-immune imbalance was not severe enough to cause the actual disease to develop. The feline AIDS is also a good example of this phenomenon.

This is probably why HIV-positive humans sometimes never develop the full AIDS disease; their endocrine-immune imbalance was not severe enough to allow the HIV virus to develop. I have successfully treated many FIV cats and also had the opportunity, through physicians, to make suggestions on testing and treating HIV and AIDS patients.

Of the few human cases that were tested, all of the patients tested positive for Plechner's Syndrome. Upon taking replacement cortisol and T3 and T4 and making sure these patients could absorb oral hormones, all improved dramatically.

CASE 20

Bleeding disorders are becoming increasingly diagnosed.

There are a number of clotting factors that can be deficient or absent, in the domino effect of clotting. The British royal family is known for their inheritance of a genetic bleeding disorder called hemophilia.

In dogs, we see a bleeding disorder called Von Willebrand Disease (VWD). This is a clotting defect, which, if not identified, can be fatal due to accidents or surgical procedures. Any puncture or cuts can lead to major hemorrhage. The VWD bleeding disorder was first identified in Doberman Pinschers.

Soon after graduation, before I really understood what VWD was, I performed an ovariohysterectomy on a young Doberman. Post-surgically, everything appeared normal. After twelve hours, the incision site started to ooze blood. X-rays and ultrasound were done immediately to make sure all ligatures of major arteries involved in the surgery were still in place and working. All the tests were negative for abdominal bleeding. Everyone involved was very concerned at a high level, and the support of the owner was greatly appreciated also.

At the time, no one was aware of VWD, and there had been no prior indication of excessive bleeding; even if a nail had been cut a little short, bleeding should have continued. In any event, after multiple injections of Vitamin K for clotting, transfusion to provide clotting factors, and an abdominal pressure wrap, the patient became normal and was sent home. I was suspicious of this clotting defect but not sure how to handle further cases.

I then decided to actually test for possible VWD patients. The disorder may have been discovered in Doberman Pinschers first, but it apparently now is found in many breeds. There often is a history of bleeding from short-cut nails, cuts, bruises, punctures, blood in urine, and bleeding at injection sites.

What I found was that this is a genetic defect. A carrier for VWD can have a blood clotting factor level down to 60 percent below normal and show no signs of excessive bleeding. Below 60 percent, often a patient may develop excessive bleeding. VWD patients can have a blood clotting factor level of 60 mg %, and within my clinical experience any dog with VWD level of 60 mg % is a carrier and never should be bred unless their mate has much higher levels otherwise this bleeding disorder will be passed on to the offspring.

I also discovered that all these patients tested positive for Plechner's Syndrome and, if identified early and placed on proper hormone therapy, the VWD factor increased to normal. I was really amazed!

Several years later I had a Doberman Pinscher presented to me with a VWD level of 20 percent. The dog had not been spayed due to these low levels. Unfortunately, the eight-year-old female Doberman had developed a mammary tumor, which needed removal, plus a complete ovariohysterectomy. No one would do the surgery for fear of having the patient bleed to death. The case was referred to me. I tested the patient and found she had Plechner's Syndrome. After proper hormonal supplementation, not only did the mammary tumor start to decrease in size since the adrenal estrogen decreased, but the VWD level increased to 90 percent. I sent the patient back to the referring veterinarian for surgical excision of the mammary tumors, ovaries, and uterus.

Fortunately, the biopsy sample was negative for any malignancy, and the patient continued her hormone therapy. She is still, at fifteen years of age, doing fine, with a normal clotting ability.

Autoimmune Hemolytic Anemia (AIHA)

This is a disease of pets that is happening more frequently now than ever. There is no recognition in the veterinary medical community that a combination of genetics, environment, aging, vaccines, stress, anesthesia, snakebites, and beestings can all reduce the ability of the body to produce enough natural cortisol to control total serum estrogen and cause the immune system to stop the abilities of these immune cells to recognize of self tissue and cease to make antibodies to many normal tissues, including red blood cells. These deregulated immune cells not only do not protect the patient, which is their intended role in immune function, but they also aggressively turn against the body itself in a highly destructive manner. These cells are not deficient by any means. They are normal, non-pathogenic immune cells. They are simply deregulated and very harmful to the patient.

The only immune deficiency is with the B cells' production of antibody. The significance of this is that when the B cells' production of the mucous membrane antibody [IgA] is below a certain level, this opens up all the areas that are normally protected by IgA to disease. This is when the respiratory tract, uro-genital tract, and digestive tract can no longer function properly to sustain normal organic function.

When the failure hits the digestive tract, malabsorption occurs through the wall of the gut. In this situation, almost no oral medication will be absorbed at the desired rates across the gut wall. Often, when a medication appears not to work, a new medication is given. What is the point, if the patient has Plechner's Syndrome and cannot absorb oral medication and nutrients across the gut wall?

As we have indicated before, there is a hormonal regulatory mechanism breakdown. We have already spoken about this hormonal regulatory mechanism that relates to a nonfunctional natural cortisol, which leads to a high total serum estrogen level, and not only a binding of the thyroid hormones but also a deregulated immune system that is now attacking the red blood cells. This is the same reason we see clotting defects with anti-platelet antibodies and why we see anti-white-cell antibodies, called lupus. When this hormonal regulatory mechanism is imbalanced, nothing in the body is really safe from the resultant deregulated immune system. Maybe the impact area is determined by genetics. I do not have the answer to this. I do wonder why some family lines seem to be prone to similar impact areas. It does begin to sound like genetics. From a clinical perspective, it has the look and feel of a genetic predisposition to certain types of organic effects when Plechner's Syndrome is evident. Even if we could diagnose the specialized gene identification in a patient, the imbalance would also need to be identified in the patient to enable physicians to make up the deficits with hormonal supplement controls, repairing the imbalances that this inherited gene has caused.

Why become a predictable statistic when you can live by something the medical profession is now beginning to realize? We know at this point that oral cortisol replacement usually will not work due to malabsorption via the gut wall, so what will work? Obviously, in the beginning of treatment, injectable cortisol must be administered. For the improved health of the patient, I have found that a combination of Vetalog and Depomedrol is the answer. The reason for using both is that the Vetalog gets into the system immediately via intramuscular injection and lasts for five to seven days, and if the Depomedrol is given in the muscle, it may take five to seven days to begin to work. Depending on how low the IgA level is, it might take two or three series of injections before oral cortisol will be available in the bloodstream via absorption via the gut. At the same time that the injectable steroid is given, thyroid hormone should be given orally. This hormone appears, because of its molecular size, to be at least partially absorbed. What is not usually realized in the medical profession is that you must not use an ongoing cortisol replacement without a thyroid hormone supplementation. The reason for this is that, without a thyroid hormone supplementation in the bloodstream, the cortisol replacement will not be completely broken down in twenty-four hours, and some cortisol from the dosage administered in the morning of the day before will remain in the bloodstream. After one to two weeks on the appropriate cortisol replacement dosage, with the daily leftover cortisol remnant of the supposed physiological dosage, it becomes a pharmacological dose and causes an overdose. These facts are not really understood very well in the medical profession.

Autoimmune Hemolytic Anemia (AIHA)

The baseline dosage rates for Vetalog and Depomedrol intramuscular injections:

- Vetalog: 0.5 milligrams per ten pounds body weight.

- Depomedrol: between 1.0 and 1.5 milligrams per pound body weight

I have noted what I feel to be a decrease in the effectiveness of the Depomedrol at the 1.0 milligrams per pound dosage that I used to use as a starting point. Therefore, I have found that I have had to at times increase the dosage up to 1.5 milligrams per pound based on the severity of the symptoms and the individual response to the injection in the animal being treated.

If more than one injection is needed to bypass the low IgA in the intestines with a combination injection, and increased thirst and appetite occurs within the first 3 to 5 days post injection, than the next injections needed should not contain Vetalog, Kenalog or Triamcinilone.

With the treatment of autoimmune hemolytic anemia, in the beginning stages huge amounts of cortisol are given (1 milligram per pound of body weight). This may be fine if the patient can absorb via the gut wall. This, hopefully, will work, and then the patient is put on a reduced amount of oral cortisol because, after all, cortisol is "bad," even though the reason the disease occurred is because the patient has an imbalance in cortisol. The treating medical professionals usually do not have a clue as to how to use cortisol safely.

There is a species variation that needs to be recognized. When using an ongoing cortisol replacement in a dog, T4 is used. In a cat, only cortisol is indicated in correcting 90 percent of the imbalances, unless feline infectious peritonitis is involved; then T4 must be given. Ninety percent of horses are required to take only T4, while humans need T3 and T4 to correct the imbalance safely.

Remember, T4 is only an inactive hormone. T3 is the active thyroid hormone. So when you go to your health care specialist, and only T4 is administered, what is the point? You now realize that imbalanced cortisol reduces the ability of T4 to be transferred to active thyroid, T3. When the total estrogen is high, then both T3 and T4 are chemically bound by the estrogenic hormones in the bloodstream. So when you are told by your health care professional that your or your pet's thyroid level is normal, you now have some questions to ask. If your health care professional doubts you or, worse, "looks down his or her nose at you," it is time to go elsewhere.

You need to remember, that whether genetic, environmental, acquired, due to aging, or for whatever reason, the prescribed hormone supplementation therapy will most likely have to be followed for life. The beauty of Plechner's Syndrome is that blood serum levels can be checked every six to twelve months to see if the natural glands were merely suppressed and not totally damaged, after the patient has been supplemented back to normal.

It is okay to try natural products if the patient is not having major problems. If the patient is having major problems, it is the veterinarian's job to get your pet "back on the fence," even with synthetics, until you have a safe opportunity to replace the synthetic supplements with holistic and homeopathic supplements. Just remember, because it is natural, it does not mean it is necessarily good for you or your pet's health. The best treatment for all patients is a combination of Eastern medicine and Western medicine. It appears that many health care professionals have "a tree" but definitely do not have the forest. Good medicine is holistic. It puts patients back to health as an entire entity. You must consider nutrition, plant-based enzymes, nutriceuticals, essential amino acids only found in foods, stress management, exercise, and all those environmental inputs that will damage the endocrine control of the immune system known as Plechner's Syndrome and cause diseases for which only the effects are treated, not the root cause.

Diabetes Mellitus

Diabetes is a very common disorder seen in pets and humans. In pets presenting with diabetes mellitus, there is often an underlying hormonal antibody imbalance—Plechner's Syndrome. This is due to the imbalanced cortisol leading to high estrogen levels in the blood stream. The elevated estrogen levels present deregulate not only the thyroid gland but also the immune cells.

Once deregulated by the excess estrogen, the thyroid cannot function well to keep up the regulator metabolism of other glands and their secretions. These imbalances now allow the deregulated immune cells to lose recognition of self tissue and self secretions (the body), and they subsequently make anti-antibodies to many matured cells and secretions in the body, including insulin.

If permanent damage has not been done to the pancreatic cells and the reregulation of the immune cells returns, then insulin production is normal and this state of diabetes no longer exists in the animal. However, if the hormonal supplementation is stopped, the diabetes state might present itself again.

It is recognized in people that the middle layer adrenal cortex works with the pancreas to keep blood sugars normal. The insulin production comes from the endocrine portion of the pancreas and helps the cells to use the glucose or blood sugar. Once blood sugar level drops, the normal cortisol helps to increase the blood sugar levels again, recreating a homeostasis. You can see where a cortisol imbalance in a person can raise havoc with trying to manage blood sugars. If this is true, then what is happening with our dogs and cats?

Almost any kind of environmental input can damage the middle layer adrenal cortex, which produces cortisol and may lead to this imbalance. Events like anesthesia, toxins, vaccines, stress, stinging insects, food impurities, and other severe diseases may lead to this hormonal regulatory mechanism breakdown. Once the total estrogen is too high, Plechner's Syndrome will begin.

What about eating plants high in a form of estrogen, like soybeans, which contains a form of estrogen called estradiol? Plant estrogens are referred to as phytoestrogens. What about estrogens coming from plastics, called xenoestrogens? It makes one wonder about bottled water in plastic. This needs to be tested for, to make sure humans and our pets are not being subjected to another form of invasive estrogen. What about plastic water pipes in the house, bringing water to you and your pets? Has this ever been tested? Total estrogen in people and pets, for the most part, are not being tested. I tried, ten years ago, to have a major metropolitan water district check for total estrogen. They obviously were not interested and did not think estrogen in drinking water was an important issue!

Many times, obesity seems to be connected to diabetes, particularly in humans. When the hormonal antibody imbalance is present, the high estrogen binding the thyroid secretions can lead to weight gain. It is a known fact that aromatase (an enzyme found in fat tissue) causes certain male and female hormones, like androgen, DHEA, and DHEAS, to be turned into total estrogen. Therefore, the heavier the patient becomes, the greater the amount of aromatase and damaging estrogen may be produced. Could this be part of the vicious cycle? Good health in people and pets comes from a normal teeter-totter effect between active cortisol and total estrogen.

Cats seem to have a little different form of diabetes mellitus than dogs and people do. In their hormonal antibody deregulation state, the high total estrogen, allowing for the deregulation of the immune cells, allows for the production of anti-antibody to insulin. If the pancreatic cells producing insulin have not been permanently damaged, then with proper hormone supplementation, the reregulated immune cells free up the insulin and the cat is no longer diabetic.

Veterinarians generally believe that if you try to regulate insulin therapy, you cannot do so if the cat is on cortisol. You can begin to see what their dilemma is. You can regulate blood glucose levels, but if you do not also regulate the hormone imbalance, often the cat will perish. In some cats, if the deregulated immune cells have permanently damaged the insulin-producing cells, then hormone and insulin therapy is indicated for the life of the cat.

Can you imagine the possible advantage to testing prospective parents and then testing their offspring to make sure this imbalance is not present in the offspring? If it is present in the parents or the offspring, then correct or control the imbalance before a disease occurs.

Prevention of a disease is always the best treatment. The hormonal antibody imbalance is the basis for many catastrophic diseases. The diseases are obviously medical effects caused by the imbalance, and not the cause. The medical practices of today, for the most part, have not kept up with today's patients or their environment.

Today, medical doctors and veterinarians believe that a cortisol replacement therapy can and will cause a state of diabetes. I believe that this is untrue; yet, as a held belief, they do not realize that a cortisol deficiency or imbalance is at the base of the problem which manifests as a diabetic condition in many patients. Now, increasingly today, many of the veterinary academics are beginning to realize specifically that regarding the possibility of steroids causing diabetes, what they are seeing in their patients is merely a side effect or manifestation of an existing hormonal imbalance in the patient. The use of lower therapeutic steroid dosages actually helps in rebalancing hormone levels and does not hurt the overall hormonal imbalance situation in their diabetic patients. It is my belief, based upon my years of experience, that if a diabetic condition does occur, not only is there a need to correct the hormonal and antibody imbalance, but there is also an emphatic need to control the insulin level imbalance directly as that is what is causing the elevated blood glucose levels in the patient. All hormone levels must be monitored and simultaneously adjusted toward normal levels at all times to fully treat the diabetic condition in the patient.

Diabetes Insipidus and Oxytocin Imbalance

[Posterior pituitary hormonal imbalance]

This is a fairly uncommon hormonal disorder associated with the posterior portion of the pituitary gland. A special anti-diuretic hormone is normally produced to reabsorb water from the small units of the kidneys to help keep the patient hydrated without experiencing dehydration problems.

Besides the obvious clinical signs of increased water intake and the associated increased urination, the hormonal disorder is usually diagnosed with urine specific gravity or density. Carefully removing water intake from the sick patient reveals that the density or specific gravity does not change. *It is always safer to take a body weight on the patient, and when the water is removed, only continue the water deprivation until the patient has lost 3 percent of his or her body weight and then restore water or IV fluids immediately.* Other diseases causing low specific gravity urine will often show an increase in the specific gravity of the urine upon water deprivation.

I offer this as a case of interest for all of you to ponder. A pregnant female Samoyed being treated in another state was carrying what appeared to be eight healthy puppies. X-rays of the uterus demonstrated healthy growing puppies. The usual gestation period for a canine mother is sixty to sixty-five days.

If the gestation period goes longer than sixty-five days, intervention is indicated. Either induce uterine contractions by giving an injection of oxytocin, another kind of posterior pituitary hormone, or perform a Cesarean section. If induction is indicated and after twenty minutes if there is no sign of uterine contractions or some sort of presentation, a C-section is in order.

I made these recommendations to the attending veterinarian, who in turn informed the owner that the Samoyed was now at sixty-five days, and action to initiate delivery of the pups was in order.

One week later, I heard from the veterinarian that the owner did not want anything invasive to be done. They decided to wait to see what would happen. They did nothing, and the mother and all eight puppies died. The attending veterinarian and owner did not understand why this occurred.

Upon questioning the attending veterinarian, I was told that the dog already had a diagnosed posterior pituitary imbalance and had been under treatment with the anti-diuretic hormones for a few years. The other posterior pituitary hormone, oxytocin, is not only necessary for milk letdown in the pregnant dog but also for uterine contractions to initiate the birthing process.

It was quite apparent this poor dog had a nonfunctional posterior pituitary gland, allowing for these disorders to occur.

Cats

We all love our cats dearly. I had a wonderful client, Roz Wheelock, who gave a cat to me, which I then gave to my son and his wife. This great cat was a Bengal named Malakai. He lived with them for many years in Hawaii. When they came to Idaho, it was to take care of me. We decided to buy a dog like they had on the mainland and then in Hawaii. My son, Jay, ran my hospital, and his wife handled the front office. This was a really great situation for me because they really cared and did a wonderful job.

When I discovered this endocrine-immune regulatory mechanism over forty years ago, which has now helped more than 120,000 cats, dogs, and humans, only my family supported me in my efforts as I tried to educate other veterinarians. After forty years of effort, I retired out of frustration. If you can, try to imagine that you have come upon and comprehended a medical mechanism that explains the cause of feline leukemia (FeLV), feline AIDS (FIV) and feline infectious peritonitis (FIP). Further, that it is possible to successfully treat cats with FeLV, with clinical 85 percent survival, on simple hormone replacement for the rest of their lives. FIV and FIP patients survive in 70 percent of the cases with similar lifelong hormone treatment, but these facts are also not recognized in my profession. I retired because no one seemed to be really interested in the answers.

Like you, I always have loved my animals, and I certainly missed them in retirement. In my practice I have actually had great animals that boarded with me that did not want to go home. I really have never been bitten by an animal because they know I would never hurt them. The three of us in Idaho procured three Fila puppies named Olive, Burly, and Jack. We knew they would grow big and strong and hopefully survive the wolves that were transplanted into Idaho. It seems like every time humans introduce nonnative species into an already damaged environment, major problems occur. The sensible thing to do is to introduce sterile individuals into the altered environment. Why not introduce spayed and neutered species first to see what impact they will have on the new environment and the other species that live there? In any event, when we took Olive in to be spayed, there was a cage of free kittens in the waiting room and they all were worth taking home. My son and I grabbed two of the little brothers wrapped in each other's arms, and we named them Bert and Ernie.

There are so many disorders in cats that can be successfully managed only if the cause is treated as well as the symptoms. Trust me, the results would be much happier for the patient as well as the owner if the cause of the symptoms is successfully treated instead of merely the symptoms. The only problem here is that you, as an owner, need to be open to a different way of thinking and believing. If you and your health care professional are achieving great results eliminating symptoms in your cat, great. However, if you are not getting the results you and your cat expected, you may want to consider a different approach to attaining good health. You may have been merely treating symptoms, not the cause of the symptoms.

Let's begin with some of the subtle indicators of an endocrine-immune imbalance in your cat. Did you ever realize that oft times, major diseases do not just happen? There is a reason the cat often develops problems. I am sure you have considered a number of reasons this is occurring. I also know that vaccines, flea deterrents, anesthesia, stress, environmental damage, and aging may be involved. Did you ever wonder why this is occurring?

Let's start with the actual mechanism that, if damaged, will definitely lead to a disease, whether minimal or catastrophic. You need to realize that the "computer chips" of the body are the adrenal glands. They lie just anterior to the kidneys. In the old days they were called suprarenal glands. The center of the gland produces adrenaline. The actual outer layer of this gland is called the cortex. The first layer of the gland helps to regulate blood pressure and electrolytes. What I want you to pay attention to is the middle layer of the adrenal cortex and the inner layer of the adrenal cortex.

This is occurring in cats because not only is there breeding for structure and color but, as mentioned above, there are environmental damages, toxins, vaccines, anesthesia, stress, and aging. What I hope to do is to help you identify why this has happened and not only show you how to control the problem but also how to prevent the problem before it occurs. Therein lies the best form of medicine.

You may also find this hard to believe, but did you ever think or realize that you produce natural cortisol from your middle adrenal cortex? Many people do not know this.

Let's look now at how this all applies to various diseases and adverse medical reactions.

FELINE RETROVIRUSES

You may not be familiar with this term, but it represents the viruses that cause feline leukemia, feline infectious anemia, and feline infectious peritonitis. All of the cats in which the regulatory mechanism breaks down, if exposed to any of these of these viruses, will usually break out with the disease. Why is this happening? All these cats will show similar test results if the tests are done correctly and the serum has been kept refrigerated from the time the sample was taken until the sample is run by the laboratory. What you will find is a cortisol imbalance evident via an elevated total estrogen level, which not only binds the thyroid hormone receptor sites but also deregulates the immune system, which simply comprises a B lymphocyte and a T lymphocyte. The B cell protects the body from invasive bacteria and is responsible for making antibodies against invading organisms, plus it is responsible for making protective antibodies against vaccines. The T cell is there to protect your cat against viruses, molds, and fungi. When these cells are deregulated, not only do they not protect your cat but they lose recognition of self breakdown tissues and thus cause major damage to healthy tissues. This is called autoimmunity. When this form of imbalance occurs, the immune system is usually thought to be deficient when it is actually in a deregulated state. The only deficiency that does actually occur during hormonal imbalance is the B cell production of antibodies.

If a kitten or cat has this hormonal imbalance, vaccinating a kitten for any of these viruses is a waste of time because of the deficiency in the numbers of B cells to create the desired immunity. Furthermore, the estrogen-bound thyroid hormones will not allow the vaccine material to break down correctly and may be perceived to be foreign substances that have now has turned into an overdose for the number of B cells present in the animal. This will give you some facts behind why vaccines are in such disfavor.

Please remember while doing replacement therapy for this hormonal imbalance that the B cell lower production of antibody, which includes the antibody that protects the mucous membranes throughout the body, is called IgA.

Once this antibody, IgA, falls below a minimum test level, the patient cannot absorb oral nutrients or replacement hormones given orally. This is why you or your cat may have experienced a stay in the hospital and, when put on IV medication or intramuscular medication, began to recover. When you were sent home on the same medication taken orally, you became sick again. The usual verbiage you will hear is, "Let's try a different medication." What is the point? If you have this endocrine-immune imbalance, the replacement therapy needs to bypass the gut totally in order to be effective. Therefore, long-acting injections must be done, or transdermal hormones used, to effectively replace the cortisol and refund the negative feedback to the pituitary, thereby reducing the total estrogen. This leads to a reregulation of the immune cells and an increasing production of IgA, which will then allow the absorption of oral nutrients and oral hormones. A partial test is run and checked every two weeks and injections given at a two-week interval. Once the IgA level is high enough again, then oral supplementation will work. Once normalized, the blood levels can be checked yearly. I have found that a very high percentage of these cases have genetic defects present along with this deregulated endocrine immune mechanism. This is one reason why holistic, homeopathic, and herbal remedies usually do not work. You can't enhance the integrity of something that is not there. Good functional hormones need to be produced and present in the body for these therapies to be beneficial. It may be worth trying once the cat is stabilized by replacing the synthetic hormones with more natural substances. The beauty of treating animals with this defect is that the blood levels present in the tests will tell you if you are proceeding in the right direction for the patient. Just remember, just because it is natural, it does not mean that it will agree with every patient and effect a cure.

In treating an FIP patient, a form of thyroid called T4 is indicated. Even though malabsorption is occurring in the gut, the molecular structure of the thyroid hormone seems to allow for sufficient absorption for therapeutic results to be achieved. As the IgA levels rise in subsequent test results, the dosage level of thyroid replacement, T4 oral hormone, needs to be lowered. Even though this may seem involved, it really is straightforward for any health care professional to do. They merely have to understand this deregulation mechanism, respect your wishes, and do what you ask for the successful treatment of your cat. Why not do the test? If the mechanism imbalance is present in the test results, either act upon it or refer to someone who will help the cat. I frequently refer my patients. If I do not know how to diagnose and treat, I refer to another doctor that has more knowledge about the condition presented than I do. When a referral will make a difference for my patient, I always make the referral.

Also realize that your vet's best information comes from you, the owner. If your veterinarian looks down his or her nose at you, doesn't listen to you, and does not want to answer your questions so you understand what he or she believes needs to be done for your cat, then move on. Egos have no place in the treatment room and can cause you to make sacrifices in your pet's health care. Remember, if you test the other cats in the family and they are negative for the virus, their endocrine-immune mechanisms are probably normal. However, if one or two of the residents in the household are positive for the virus, then check the mechanism to see if there is an imbalance. If there is an imbalance, it needs to be corrected via replacement hormone therapy before the medical effect occurs. If the cat or cats are normal with the mechanism when tested, then watch them yearly to make sure as they age there is not a weakening of this regulatory mechanism. Remember, no matter what you have been told or heard, a cat that has the disease can, once the endocrine-immune regulatory mechanism is rebalanced, not only shed the virus but also cease to be a carrier.

GINGIVAL FLARE

When you are purchasing a kitten or rescue a stray or already have your good buddy or buddies at home, it is always important to identify an imbalance before a medical effect occurs. The beauty of this mechanism is that it not only helps correct many catastrophic diseases in your cat but can also predict and prevent diseases from occurring. Therein lies your best treatment. A gingival flare can be identified as a slight to major red line or area where the gum reflects upon the tooth enamel. This may be seen in 70 percent of cats and represents an IgA deficiency due to Plechner's Syndrome. The test should be done on all cats and can be done in a kitten as early as eight weeks of age. If the kitten is small, it is best to wait until the kitten is four months of age. Only a partial test is indicated. This test will only check cortisol, total estrogen, and thyroid hormones, T3 and T4. If an imbalance is found, the rebalance correction therapy needs to be started immediately. This will stop any future problems from occurring, and it also makes sure that the reduced IgA levels due to the imbalance do not hamper growth due to malabsorption via the gut. This malabsorption due to the imbalance not only restricts a lack of essential growth nutrients from the gut, but it can cause further damage to the glands that produce management hormones that regulate the immune cells.

Unfortunately, many cats have had to go through multiple teeth cleanings for their inflamed gums. Many times this condition seems to improve with a total tooth extraction. The food buildup around the tooth will now not challenge the IgA deficiency as badly since there is less food retention and less uncontrolled bacteria to invade the deficiency in the gums.

Since this IgA deficiency will be found throughout all the mucous membrane-containing systems in the body, there appears to be a genetic input as far as to where the impacted area will occur. Sometimes, accompanying the gingival flare you may see chronic respiratory problems, chronic urinary tract problems, digestive tract problems, or chronic eye and ear problems.

SKIN SENSITIVITIES

If your cat is checked by your health care professional and external parasites and fungi are found but no medical treatment will eliminate the problem, you may want to have the endocrine-immune panel (EI-1 test) done.

Most skin diseases are caused by this regulatory mechanism imbalance. This is definitely not to say that you should not let your practitioner treat the medical effects, but identifying the root cause will usually stop the problem from recurring. With the regulatory mechanism breakdown, often topical and oral or injectable antibiotics will help for a while, but the skin problem will usually return. Have you ever wondered why this happens? With the animal in regulatory imbalance, there is very little immune protection available; therefore, the normal staphylococcus bacteria are now able to grow in greater numbers in this unchallenged environment. In the wall of the bacteria, there is an allergen called a mucopolysaccharide. With the increase of the total bacteria count, and therefore the increase in the amount of allergen, the skin problems worsen during the duration of the regulatory mechanism imbalance.

Once the antibiotic works, and the bacteria and their allergens are reduced, the skin problem gets better. That is, until the regrowth of the bacteria recurs as the antibiotic metabolizes out of the host animal's system. However, when the same antibiotic is consistently used to treat this same condition while a regulatory mechanism breakdown is present, the bacteria are not really challenged by the deregulated immune cells. At such times, the bacteria have a better chance of developing a resistance to that antibiotic. While this is occurring, the regulatory mechanism imbalance usually worsens. As this happens and the total estrogen rises, the IgA level throughout the body decreases. When the level of this antibody goes below a certain level on testing, malabsorption occurs, so even if you were satisfied with assuming the skin could not get any better, the antibiotic that had helped previously no longer can because now it cannot be absorbed through the gut wall. Injectable and transdermal antibiotics might work for a time, but usually they, too, will cause enough bad changes in the good resident bacteria in the body that other medical problems will usually develop.

URINE-SPRAYING FEMALES

Have you ever wondered why your female cat is acting like a non-neutered male cat and appears to be marking her territory? With the mechanism imbalance, the unresponsive cortisol is either too deficient to respond to the pituitary or is in a form the pituitary gland does not recognize. So the feedback mechanism is damaged. The pituitary gland keeps producing its hormone, adrenal-corticotrophin hormone (ACTH). The only other layer in the body that can respond to ACTH is the inner layer of the adrenal cortex. Guess what? We now know where the high levels of estrogen come from. But did you know a large quantity of male hormone is also produced, called androgen? When the mechanism is imbalanced, this can occur, causing your female cat to act like a male. This often corrects itself and is not a learned behavior. If the problem continues, it may be time to see an animal behaviorist. Definitely do this testing before you change your carpets [A little bad humor.]

CANCER OR UNCONTROLLED TISSUE GROWTH

Whether this occurs in cats, dogs, horses, or people, they all have a hormonal imbalances; this is known after measuring levels in over two hundred thousand cases. This no longer can be considered research. These are proven facts. You and your pet definitely do not want to become a statistic due to medical ignorance. Always remember, it is better to live with a new hope than die by the book. All cancer patients have Plechner's Syndrome. The effects must be treated, but cause needs to be funded, also. As chemotherapy, radiation therapy, and anesthesia are done for excision, the patient must be watched for any hormonal changes that may need to be funded due to the Plechner's Syndrome in order to keep the patient normal.

PERSONALITY DEFECTS

Did you ever wonder why your cat is not more social? Is it really a lack of socialization since you have had this cat since it was a kitten? Why then, when your cat comes up to you for a little love and you pat your cat on the back, does it turn around and bite you? Do you really accept this as something cats just do? Why is this often accepted as the norm when it definitely is not? All of these previous signs relate to Plechner's Syndrome. All these problems can be diagnosed and treated if they are symptoms of Plechner's Syndrome.

Plechner's Syndrome relates to many personality changes that can be very subtle to very overt. The following are examples of this. Has your cat ever come up to you purring for a little attention and when you started to pet him or her on the back they would turn around and either scratch or bite you? This is very common with this Plechner's Syndrome patients. Apparently there is an inflammation of the nerves to the back called neuritis. When the area is touched, the cat will react because it hurts. There are usually no signs of this reflected on the skin. A not-quite-so-enjoyable event blessed my presence one day. My partner asked me to see this Abby cat that I did not know was fractious. I introduced myself to the owner, and she then opened up the carrier and here was the patient trying to strike at me. I do love cats, and even the toughest of cats usually yield to me; however, this cat was going to eat me alive. Sorry, I had no salt and pepper so that I might taste better. The owner said, "Go ahead and pull Ralph out because he is only bluffing." I said, "He is not bluffing, and if I get him out he cannot be controlled. It is not fair to get Ralph this upset. Why not let me send you home with a mild sedative to give to Ralph in two days and come back to see his regular vet." The owner became highly irate and said I was chicken s&*t. I said, "You're absolutely correct." She proceeded to take Ralph out of his box, and Ralph severely bit and scratched her. She was bleeding like a stuck pig. I wanted to attend to her wounds, but she said no and asked to leave the room as Ralph, with his ears flat to his head and with now-almond-shaped eyes and bristled tail, began to stalk me. Fortunately, there were side doors at each end of this long room, so I bailed quickly. By now, the entire hospital was standing by to see how Ms. Siegfried and Roy would fare. Soon after, a weakened cry for help came from the exam room and, as we peeked in, Ralph's owner was hunched over with Ralph's claws in her back. We decided to rush the situation with two cardboard boxes. One person came from each side of the exam room. We scooped Ralph off the owner's back, dumped him in his carrier, and instructed the owner go see her physician for some antibiotics and a tetanus vaccine. Ralph's future gave my partner something to think about.

Why, when your cat possibly gets stressed or eats a new food or snack, does it have a seizure? It is of interest to note that since phenobarbital is most often used in a cat with idiopathic epilepsy that the serum phenobarbital levels often remain low, so the dosage level of the drug is raised to reach proper blood serum levels for seizure management. You already know, because of Plechner's Syndrome, the decreased IgA level has reduced the absorption of the phenobarbital, and when the hormone supplementation is done to correct Plechner's Syndrome, an overdose of the phenobarbital is absorbed and the patient may become overmedicated, leading to a loss of consciousness. This also holds true for diabetics because as Plechner's Syndrome is corrected, the immune cells become reregulated and recognize insulin as self tissues. All of a sudden, the anti-insulin antibodies decrease in number, and with this in combination with the injectable insulin, you are now faced with an overdose of insulin. This causes the blood sugar to fall precipitously, and the patient becomes wobbly, then has a seizure and dies. You must always keep honey or Karo syrup on hand to give to your cat if you think this is happening. Remember, you can always reregulate your cat if the blood glucose is temporarily too high from the glucose supplement you have given. But if you guess wrong and do not give the sugar supplement, you could watch your cat die.

FOOD SENSITIVITY

Cats can have food sensitivities, but the actual typical clinical signs seem to be different. Just a simple note: remember that humans can speak and discuss their problems, but since animals cannot speak, we rely on signs.

Often, with a cat, when a certain food causes vomiting, it is due to an inflamed stomach caused by Plechner's Syndrome, which has produced an irritable bowel syndrome. It may cause not only vomiting and diarrhea but also malabsorption of nutrients and drugs through the gut wall. Many times by correcting the hormonal imbalance, the same food will be tolerated. However, with Plechner's Syndrome, there is very little if any protection of the secondary organs that may be affected by this hormonal imbalance. There can be liver disease due to Plechner's Syndrome because the food allergens can go to the liver for processing and breakdown. Breakdown cannot occur there because of Plechner's Syndrome and the fact that the high estrogen level can cause inflammation of the lining cells of the hepatic arteries, leading to an abnormal increase in the release of hepatic enzymes, indicating acute and possible long-term damage to the liver. What I believe is more damaging is the inflammation of the pancreas that can lead to an insufficiency in its endocrine function, insulin production, plus a possible exocrine deficiency in the production of the digestive enzyme called trypsin. I have seen a number of cases in which a food sensitivity has caused a lack of insulin, and a state of diabetes resulted. Once the food sensitivity issue is settled, the problem will normalize itself if permanent damage has not been done. If this has happened, then insulin is indicated, plus not only hormone replacement to correct the Plechner's Syndrome defects indicated, but also a trypsin replacement so that the patient can absorb nutrients and the oral hormonal replacements.

HYPERTHYROIDISM

Present-day practices diagnose hyperthyroidism by a high T4 level. The practitioners of today do the T4 test and palpate the neck area to see if there is a nodule present. If so, a chemical is used to destroy the thyroid tissue, not unlike radiation therapy done on people for enlarged thyroid. Without doing testing for both T4 and T3, you do not know if there is a tumor of the thyroid. Most health care professionals rely on the T4 values alone. You now know that with a Plechner's Syndrome patient, a lack of natural cortisol will stop transference of storage T4 to active T3. Why not test for both hormones before you kill your patient? What about high total estrogen acting to bind both T3 and T4? All these levels need to be checked in diagnosing Plechner's Syndrome before you possibly "pull the trigger."

I have the veterinary lab I use listed on my website, and I have worked with physicians using Quest labs. The problem I have encountered with getting other labs interested in running this test is that they need to know how many of these tests they need to run to make a profit.

Elimination Diets

What does this really mean? If you really suspect your dog or cat has some sort of food sensitivity, then what should you do? Certainly check with your health care professional first to make sure that a particular food was properly formulated and does not contain products that might cause serious health problems. Unfortunately, we have seen much of this over the past few years. If the food you are feeding is a proper food formulation and your pet is still showing signs of food sensitivity, then it is likely that your pet has an endocrine-immune imbalance. Remember, the immune mechanism imbalance occurs before the patient begins to react. Often, it is the old diet that deregulated cells have been exposed to long enough to cause a reaction. Please do not keep trying new diets because, with this imbalance, the immune cells will eventually react to all of the foods. You may find your pet in that category where there are no foods left on earth that your pet can tolerate. This same predicament can occur in people as well. If you have tried all the recommendations from all the food manufacturers and nothing positive happened, there definitely is a way to actually solve this problem.

After fifty years of applied practice, I clearly understand that the foods I have to have for my patients must contain fewer types of food allergens and at the same time make sure that the food formulations are proper to avoid new food sensitivities in the future. So what is the next step for you to do?

Changing the food might be a temporary answer, but this may not be the solution. If the food being fed to your pet works for you, great. Keep feeding it. But just remember, foods do change. The foods that I created to help pets were designed to help me decide if there was a food sensitivity present. I found there were. But many years ago, my Nature's Recipe and the IVD diets were copied by many pet food manufacturers. This was a good thing for the pets. It helped clean up the pet food market. Owners were now reading the labels and buying only those foods they could trust. But can you really trust the label and know it represents what is actually in that food? I could not believe this, and that is one reason I created my own foods—if an animal had a reaction to my food, I knew exactly what was in the food. This would help me do an elimination study on my patient to determine the food that was eliciting the sensitivity. Eventually,

Nature's Recipe and the IVDs were sold. I have to say, sadly, that the ingredients in those foods have been changed. There are still pet foods available that have an ingredient list that is close to my original formulas. Unfortunately, you will have to seek these out yourself. The diets are now different. I had hoped that I had set a better standard for pet foods but obviously not. Since I have retired, the pet food manufacturers have gone to playing the commodities as part of their pet food ingredients from a financial standpoint. If these changes are not listed on the label, you could innocently give to your pet an unlisted food ingredient that could end in tragedy.

So, what do you want to do? If you and your pet are happy with what is being fed, that is good. If, however, you are frustrated like most of us are, let's continue on. What do we do next? I think the future is evident. You need to cook for your pet, but only foods that are safe enough to feed to your family. After all, your pet is part of your family.

Let's begin with a simple, temporary diet that hopefully agrees with your pet. I would suggest using only one source of protein and one source of carbohydrate. Even doing this, I found that in time, if the protein and possibly the carbohydrate were not rotated at a two- to three-month interval, sensitivities may occur due to this immune mechanism breakdown. The main purpose for using this kind of select food was not only to identify a food sensitivity but also to remove a variable from this equation that is dominant. You now need to have the endocrine-immune panel done. Once correctly funded by your health care professional, you can then begin to add foods back. You need to know what foods have caused sensitivities in your pet in the past. The reason for this is that many health care professionals believe that if you purge the offensive foods for you and your pet for a few weeks or more, you will occasionally be able to feed them to you or your pet without a reaction. Personally, I have found just the opposite. I usually observed a more severe reaction than ever before. Remember, the immune cells do not forget or forgive. This is why not treating the deregulated immune mechanism and merely trying new foods can only lead you and your pet into a total food catastrophe. This means the immune cells will react to everything. You do not want this to happen to either one of you.

Elimination Diets

After creating the first commercial vegetarian pet foods for the world, I realized that many of the dogs and cats that ate my vegetarian diet began to develop food sensitivities. I now realize that the problem developed from the soy in the food that was naturally high in phytoestrogens. I created the first lamb and rice diets plus many other formulations for dogs and cats. One nice factor I found with the lamb was that lamb tallow was a natural preservative. I had hoped the other pet food manufacturers could relate to this. Unfortunately, they kept using their chemical preservatives, like BHA, BHT, and ethoxiquin. After a period of time, our pets developed sensitivities to lamb, chicken, rice, etc. I again was forced to develop a new food with limited ingredients that many pets had not been exposed to; hence, the beginning of Innovative Veterinary Diets. The proteins used were venison, rabbit, duck, and fish. I used white potatoes as the carbohydrate. I was the first to add eight hundred milligrams of taurine to all of the cat foods I created in order to avoid causing an enlargement of the cats' hearts, called cardiomyopathy. For your own information, taurine occurs in high amounts in chicken hearts, which are usually included as a byproduct in other cat foods. The manufacturers producing these cat foods unknowingly avoided the development of cardiomyopathy due to the natural taurine contained in the chicken hearts.

Now pet food manufacturers include all kinds of additives into their foods. You have to worry sometimes because that additive might be harmful to one animal and not to another. You may also wonder if many of these additives are destroyed during the heating process for the food ingredients. Possibly they are mixed in after the heating process is done, but then how can they be certain they are getting an equal amount of the additive throughout the entire mix? While developing all these diets, I was able to find the immune regulatory mechanism in the pet that allowed this food sensitivity to occur.

The next step is to have an Endocrine-Immune Panel 1 test run on the animal. Then, begin an elimination diet that agrees with your pet while you are waiting for the blood test results. If you do not begin with a limited antigen, then the following hints might help you pick the proper diet. The longer the label is on the pet food, the worse the diet is, because good nutrition is simple. The first three ingredients on the label are 90 percent of that diet. When you are told that this really is a meaty treat, and beef is the seventh item listed on the ingredient list, this means the bull walked by the barn and waved. Also remember, tomato pumice is thought to be a better roughage than beet pulp. This is kind of what I have learned over the years. Pet food may have changed over the years, but I am always ready to learn and use new food concepts if it will make a difference for my patients.

If you already know my recommendation might be a problem for your pet, you should definitely go in a different direction. If you ever need help, I can always be consulted on my website under Contacts. It would be best to begin with only two additives, which you can do from home. Let's try one protein and one carbohydrate. I have found in dogs, with cottage cheese and boiled white potatoes, a one-to-four ratio might be a place to begin. With cats, you might try a protein the cat likes with a carbohydrate like potato or ground peas or squash in the same one-to-four ratio.

Cottage Cheese and Potato Replacement Diet.

One part cottage cheese to four parts boiled white potatoes is the ratio.

The amount fed will vary with each patient. It usually is around a cup per ten lbs of body weight AM and PM.

Please do not compare yourself to your pet. Yes, I realize that milk products in humans can be not only allergenic but are also mucous-producing. Please also remember that there are species variations. If the cottage cheese and white potato diet works for one week, then we move on. Next, add another protein, possibly chicken. It is very important to add only one new ingredient for your pet to eat in an elimination diet every seven days.

The thing that seems to be the most confusing for pet owners is realizing that a food reaction can be delayed. What does this mean? Each time you add a new food to a specialized diet, you not only need to use a small amount of the food to reduce a possible reaction to that food, but also realize that a delayed reaction may occur on up to the seventh day after feeding. So many times, I have spoken with people who have said, "I did not give anything different to my pet." My question then is, "Did you give anything different in the last seven days?" Usually, the answer is, "I did give a small snack. That could not have mattered." It does matter.

I hope none of have you have been to a cocktail party, as I was, where someone was allergic to egg whites. A wonderful salad was served, and a tiny amount of mayonnaise was included in the salad dressing. If the paramedics had not been down the street, a woman would have died. Trust me, if there is a food sensitivity, the immune cells will remember, and if the reaction is severe enough, you just may lose your pet. Someone who meant well and who just does not understand is usually the culprit. With modern inbred dogs and cats, you do not want a well-meaning relative or friend causing a catastrophe for you and your pet. The statement usually is, "I really did not know, and I am really sorry." Their intentions will never justify their well-meaning actions. Sometimes it safer to confine your pet when visitors arrive or when you and your family sit down to eat, especially if you have children. This may seem unfair for the pet, but it sure beats the alternative!

Once again I will repeat myself: if you purge your or your pet's system of any foods, like beef, etc., that you and your pet cannot tolerate, if you try the food after a given period time, you may sustain a very severe reaction. Do not do this to yourself or your pet. Once you have the endocrine-immune imbalance, the deregulated immune cells that were allowed to make sensitivities against these foods will never forget. They are a lot like elephants. And if you believe that "a little bit will not hurt," check on the Internet with people who gave a piece of "well-meaning" bacon to their pets and had their precious pets die within six hours with a terminal pancreatic necrosis. Trust me, in fulfilling your need to be someone of value to the pet by sneaking snacks under the kitchen table, you just may have cost your best friend his or her life. Feeding the wrong food to an imbalanced pet can be lethal.

Anti-Aging

Supplements, good nutrition, and exercise are highly important in slowing down the aging process, but none of these are more important than the homogeneity of the endocrine system and its regulation of the immune cells, which hopefully will protect the body.

When an imbalance occurs between natural, active cortisol and total estrogen, not only are the thyroid hormones bound, but total slowdown of metabolism can also occur. When this happens, breakdown products, toxins, etc, are not eliminated or properly broken down within a twenty-four-hour period, but remain in the body to kill vital cells needed for its healthy maintenance.

This is one reason normal cells cannot live out their normal life span of one hundred twenty days and often perish within ninety days. You can begin to see that there may be a 25 to 30 percent hastening of cellular death, contributing to early aging of the person or pet in question. The lack of immune regulation due to hormonal imbalances further leads to the immune cells losing the ability to recognize self tissue. A further reason for early aging is due to these "immune soldiers" having a better chance of attacking the person or pet's own tissues. This condition is often referred to as autoimmunity.

To determine if this is occurring and to prevent early aging, certain body fluid component measurements need to be made. Currently, only partial tests are regularly carried out to measure estrogen. Total estrogen must be measured in both sexes. In males, only estradiol is usually measured. In females, only the three ovarian estrogens are usually measured. Why, then, in my spayed females that have no ovaries, can the total estrogen be high if there is this endocrine regulatory mechanism imbalance present? Obviously, there are other sources of estrogen in the patients that are not being measured. Besides the usually recognized estrogen sources, there may be large amounts of adrenal estrogen, there may be phytoestrogens from plant or vegetable sources, and plastic may contain xenoestrogens. Do you think that the switching from copper water pipes to plastic water pipes might possibly be a significant reason there has been an increase in cancer throughout our nation? [Ed. Dr. Plechner shares his concerns about the integrity and safety of our water supply and food supply with many scientists around the world. You can read more here in this publication of the American Chemical Society. http://pubs.acs.org/cen/coverstory/87/8735cover.html.]

There may also be some concern about municipal water sources that we drink from that have not been tested for estrogens yet. If antibiotics can show up in the ground water, estrogens might, too, for the simple example as being due to people flushing estrogen supplements down the toilet.

Last, but not least, would we expect any female patient, whether a person or a pet, to take any estrogen supplement without first doing a test for total estrogen? These all play a part in the total estrogen picture. With high estrogen binding the available thyroid hormones, the estrogenic effects become even worse because the slowed metabolism in the liver due to the hypothyroid status further reduces the breakdown of the total serum estrogens.

Once you have an accurate total estrogen, how do you determine what has occurred with the immune cells? The antibody production by one type of immune cell (B cell) will determine if other immune cells (T cells) will protect the body or turn against it. With proper hormone supplementation, you not only normalize the hormones, but you can normalize the activity of both the B and T cells. This further means that each patient can be solely titrated to determine what his or her specific hormonal replacement needs will be to normalize B cell antibody production. [Ed. What Dr. Plechner has learned over the years is that when a hormonal imbalance exists, the numbers and functions of both the B and T cells of the immune systems change, more often than not, to the bad rather than good. Numbers of these essential immune cells drop, and they often become bad actors in the immune function. This is only now becoming a topic of discussion and research in the field of immunology. Dr. Plechner does not pretend to fully comprehend the mechanism. He simply knows that it exists and has learned how to safely and effectively restore both the endocrine and immune systems to balance and function.]

Anti-Aging

Over the years, I have had the privilege of treating several large breeds: Great Danes, Irish wolfhounds, Newfoundland Retrievers, St. Bernards, and Great Pyrenees. It has always been assumed that these large breeds naturally die early in life, by the time they are five to seven years of age. Could this, however, be a form of early aging?

Even with proper nutrition, proper supplements, and proper exercise, the five- to seven-year time frame still exists. This is not to say that the above factors are not important, but what it may say is that we need to look elsewhere for another reason for this shorter life span. There is another reason. By measuring the necessary serum levels to test for the presence of an imbalanced hormonal-antibody regulatory mechanism in a six-month-old large or giant breed, if there is an imbalance and it is controlled, I have been able to markedly extend the lives of my patients.

In my experience it is not unusual to have healthy Great Danes live to fifteen to sixteen years of age; Irish wolfhounds to twelve to fourteen years; Newfoundland Retrievers to fifteen to seventeen years; and St. Bernards and Great Pyrenees to fourteen to fifteen years of age.

Actually, this test not only helps in diagnosing early aging but also helps prevent medical disorders that will occur if there is a regulatory mechanism imbalance (Plechner's Syndrome). Remember this: the cause will almost always precede the effect.

Pets and people are definitely similar, if not the same, when it comes to early aging.

Contaminated Water

Is America's water poisoning you and your pet? Many people, including some scientists, are beginning to think, perhaps so.

Almost daily, we are becoming more aware of many problems with our public and private water supplies. Even in north Idaho, where I was living for a time with my son, there are contaminates that are very specific to that area due to mining operations. There, the runoff products from the mining operations go directly into the streams and percolate into the groundwater. *National Geographic* magazine has created a list of the five most beautiful lakes in the world. Three are located in Idaho. They are Coeur d'Alene, Pend Oreille, and Priest Lake. These lakes exist today as examples of man's lack of concern for his environment. We have dumped mining end products into these beautiful lakes by way of formerly pristine streams and rivers. Now, these lakes have turned into toxic waste dumps from which we and our pets drink water and eat fish. We do not know how this will affect our lives. Lead, mercury, and chlorinated hydrocarbons like DDT are now widely identified in our food chain along with other residues of other toxic chemicals, pharmaceuticals, and pesticides. I remember back in the mid-1960s when I was in vet school at the University of California at Davis; when we would drive into West Sacramento, there were signs on the bridge stating, "If you are pregnant, DO NOT EAT the fish." Probably, they referred to our old long-term enemy, mercury.

I wrote an article a few years ago for the *Journal of Toxicology* that now appears in my Compendium. It describes how often all these toxic products, including anti-flea products, can cause Plechner's Syndrome by directly affecting the middle layer of the adrenal cortex and altering its production of natural cortisol. When this occurs, the total free serum estrogen increases and can cause catastrophic diseases. As the elevated serum levels of total free estrogen bind the thyroid hormones, the metabolism of those organs, which are meant to detoxify our bodies of any contaminant, cannot eliminate toxins efficiently. The toxins not only make the body generally suffer, but the liver and kidney tissues specifically are damaged and cannot neutralize the toxins effectively. This damage, over time, will kill the patient.

There have been reports of sick and dying Beluga whales. Concurrently, young polar bears are having a problem reaching normal size, and upon being examined, one small cub carried fourteen different chemicals in its body.

We know what the water districts and other governmental agencies are checking for when they test our potable water supplies. What about damaging agents that are not being checked for? Who is checking to see if they are present in our water supply? Just recently the agencies have found antibiotics in potable water supplies. What about other medicinal drugs and hormones?

I personally worry about estrogens in our water supply. Why not check more broadly for estrogenic compounds? I know how dangerous estrogen supplements can be, especially since the health care professionals are only measuring ovarian estrogen in females and estradiol in males. What about adrenal estrogen? How about including plant estrogens, called phytoestrogens? How about estrogens that come from plastics, called xenoestrogens? Why not make sure you are not getting estrogen from plastic containers? Why not check and make sure we are not making our population sick by dosing them with estrogenic compounds? We must try our very best not to add to the problems that already exist in our pets and our own bodies.

A Summary of the Medical and PhD Endocrine Literature

This is a summary of various endocrine secretions and their possible effects that may relate to veterinary endocrinology.

ELEVATED ESTROGEN CAUSING THE PRODUCTION OF A REVERSE T3 STATUS

The elevated adrenal estrogen can cause the production of a reverse T3 does bind the T3 receptor sites.

When does this occur?

This can occur for a number of reasons. If there is a deficient, bound, or defective cortisol being produced by the middle layer adrenal cortex, the pituitary gland will produce excess ACTH, which will lead to an elevated adrenal estrogen.

The ingestion of medications and other sources in foods, plastics, and chemicals may lead to elevated exogenous estrogen that also will allow for the production of a reverse T3. Also, the cortisol imbalance impairs the transference of storage thyroid, T4, to active thyroid, T3.

The literature further suggests that the overproduction of active cortisol also causes the production of a reverse T3. This might explain why there is hair loss and further elevation of cortisol because, with the production of a reverse T3, the thyroid, being bound, slows the metabolism of the liver for cortisol breakdown and of the kidney for excretion.

This also results in a lower body temperature, which, in turn, slows down the function of many enzymes in the body, causing a state of hypothyroidism.

THYROID BINDING GLOBULIN (TBG)

TBG binds thyroid hormone that is circulating. It is one of three proteins that is a carrier for T3 and T4 in the bloodstream. It occurs only in small amounts, but does carry most of the T4 in the serum. It is produced in the liver and has only one binding site for T3 and T4.

The testing of TBG many times may not be very useful because TBG production can be modified by other factors including estrogen, corticosteroids, and liver disease.

When estrogen levels are too high, the TBG will bind T3 and T4 and cause an increase in thyroid stimulating hormone to cause more release of T3 and T4. Conversely, in the presence of corticosteroids, the TBG will be lowered, and therefore the total thyroid hormone, which is free and bound, will be lowered. This may be part of the reason why true Cushing syndrome, which causes the excess production of active cortisol, does cause a state of hypothyroidism that may completely mimic true hypothyroidism.

THYROID-STIMULATING HORMONE (TSH)

TSH is produced in the anterior pituitary gland and regulates the function of the thyroid gland. Therefore, TSH regulates T3 and T4. When their levels decrease, there is a feedback that is stimulated that goes to the hypothalamus, causing a release of thyrotropin-releasing hormone (TRH). It, in turn, is transported down to the anterior pituitary to stimulate the release of TSH.

If TSH, T3, and T4 are all elevated, or deficient, the problem may lie with the pituitary gland itself and may be due to a pituitary tumor or a thyroid hormone resistance.

If the TSH is high and the T3 and T4 are low, then the disorder is probably in the thyroid gland itself due to a true hypothyroidism or to an autoimmune thyroid disorder called Hashimoto's disease. This also may be true for a low TSH and high T3 and T4.

WHAT ARE THE CAUSES OF AN ENLARGED THYROID GLAND, REFERRED TO AS GOITER?

A deficiency in iodine can lead to a lack of thyroid hormone production. This lack of hormone production may lead to a feedback deficit to the anterior pituitary gland. This can lead to an elevation in TSH, which in turn causes the thyroid to enlarge, resulting in an endemic colloid goiter.

Many years ago, the Great Lakes were known as the Goiter Belt. This occurred because the soil around the Great Lakes was deficient in iodine. In the late 1930s or early 1940s, Morton Salt Company began to iodize its salt for this very problem.

Also, there are certain foods that contain isoflavones that block an enzyme called thyroid peroxidase, which is responsible for iodine uptake by the thyroid. Soy products may be the culprit.

There is a second group of foods that should be avoided, if you or your dog are suffering from hypothyroidism. This group of foods is referred to as the cruciferous food family. This family includes Brussels sprouts, cabbage, mustard, rutabagas, kohlrabi, and turnips. This family contains isothiocyanates, which have the same action as the isoflavones.

THE EFFECTS OF T3 (TRIIODOTHYRONINE)

It increases the basal metabolic rate and the oxygen and energy consumption of the body.

PROTEIN

It increases the rate of not only protein synthesis but also the breakdown and utilization by the body. The ratio here cannot be more protein breakdown than protein synthesis. Herein lie many diseases.

GLUCOSE

It increases the rate of breakdown of storage sugars in the body to usable glucose for the body and the cells. Most of the storage glucose, called glycogen, can be stored in the liver. If liver disease is present, then conversion disorders could lead to episodes of low blood sugar. The T3 also potentiates the effect of insulin. You can see some real reasons why a state of hypoglycemia may occur.

LIPIDS

T3 stimulates the breakdown of cholesterol but can also increase the number of receptor sites for low-density lipids that need to remain low for good health.

T3 also increases the blood circulation, called cardiac output, of the heart. It is involved with increasing systolic blood pressure and decreasing diastolic blood pressure. This may be a part of high blood pressure disorders.

T3 is important in the development of most of the systems in the body like the skeletal system, respiratory system, nervous system, and much more. It is also very important to make sure the patient does not have an elevated blood pressure, because if this is the case, prescribing a thyroid hormone could elevate the patient's blood pressure high enough to cause a stroke or a heart attack.

I think you can see how involved these systems are and how they may play into major disorders if not in a balanced state. I think it also tells us how naive we are when taking hormones and supplements. We need to bring our disorders back into sync without further unbalancing an already damaged system.

EUTHYROID (or, NONTHYROIDAL ILLNESS SYNDROME)

This is a state of hypothyroidism that may be caused by poor nutrition including starvation, systemic infections, surgery, heart attacks, transplantation procedures, chemotherapy, and probably any severe illness.

In veterinary practice, this is viewed as just part of the disease that is being treated. It is often assumed that the thyroid function will return as soon as the disease has been controlled.

I have always tried to supply thyroid hormone during this time to help the patient heal, and then after a proper amount of healing has occurred, to do a blood test to make sure the thyroid is again functioning. This helps make sure this state of euthyroid does not remain due to a permanently damaged thyroid gland.

GLUCOCORTICOIDS

High-level active cortisol, whether exogenous or endogenous, may cause a profound effect on thyroid hormone production.

The effects that occur may lead to a low serum T4, normal free T3, low serum T3, high rT3, and low normal TSH levels. The glucocorticoids can also inhibit the uptake of radioiodine and may be used in patients with a hyperthyroid state to reduce T4, T3, and thyroglobulin release.

Of interest also is that many patients who have a cortisol deficiency may have signs of hypothyroidism. This state of hypothyroidism often resolves itself upon administration of active cortisol. It is thought that this occurs because the cortisol reregulates the TSH secretion, or if there is an autoimmune thyroiditis, the cortisol reregulates the immune system to not make antibodies to thyroid tissue.

Genetic History of Pets and Wildlife

In the beginning, when humans discovered that pets might have a function that served them well, man decided to use these animals for his own benefit, often altering them in a genetically predetermined manner.

Unfortunately, as man modified animals, other sublethal and lethal genetic defects also accompanied this genetic modification that was deemed to be desirable.

During the early twentieth century, ranchers decided to breed a smaller collie so that more animals could be carried in the back of ranchers' trucks to work their cattle.

The Germans decided to crop Doberman Pinschers' ears so the ears stood erect. It was believed that this would allow the dogs to hear better while on patrol or on guard.

The firemen found Dalmatians that seemed not to mind the high-pitched sirens of the fire engines, so the dogs could ride along as mascots without getting upset. It worked well because most of the Dalmatians were deaf. The firemen discovered this, and it served their needs, but they had very little to do with the development of this genetic defect.

German Shepherds were bred with sloping backs, somewhat like the backs of hyenas. This was more of a designer dog and was apparently more appealing to man. Accompanying these changes, hip dysplasia raised its ugly head!

In 1967, I was given the opportunity to see many X-rays of German dogs. I could see the radiological changes that had begun to occur. However, the Germans simply decided to run the dogs behind their bicycles for ten miles, and if the dog did not limp, this was deemed to be a healthy dog with no signs of hip dysplasia. The radiological changes were ignored and thought to be insignificant. Today, we all know this was not the case.

At this same time, some major breeders of German Shepherds in this country were trying to buy healthy breed stud dogs from the Germans. In reviewing these X-rays, they saw that all the dogs had early signs of hip dysplasia. This was definitely not breeding stock for the future.

Often you will find the beginning genetic defect in one breed, but eventually most breeds may develop the same genetic defects based on breeding practices for structure alone.

Over time, collies were bred for longer noses, with smaller, narrower heads. This was the beginning of PRA (progressive retinal atrophy). This syndrome causes sight impairment. There are different degrees of impairment. The syndrome began with an increased tortuosity of the retinal blood vessels. This was diagnostic, and the breeders were told that even though there is no sight deficiency, the gene was still there. As PRA progressed, not only did the vascular changes occur, but areas of retinal detachment occurred, called ectasia. Ectasia refers to the detachment of the retina from the inside of the back of the actual globe.

As a sophomore at University of California at Davis, School of Veterinary Medicine, I was on call for the veterinary clinic on this one particular weekend that I recall. I hope you realize that Lassie was actually one of seven Laddies.

The owner and trainer of the Laddies traveled at this time to various shopping malls in order to have his "Lassies" perform super stunts. In West Sacramento, the owner put on his show in the parking lot of a supermarket. He had Lassie climb a ladder and jump into his arms. Lassie missed his arms and hit the asphalt.

Fortunately, upon physical examination, she seemed fine; there were no fractures. However, upon examining the eyes, I found this strange increase in the tortuosity of the retinal vessels crossing the lens of the eye, the retina was missing pigment, and the underlying pigment of the choroid layer looked like tiger stripes. This was the beginning of progressive retinal atrophy, referred to as PRA. This was the first time that I had seen this disease, and this was the summer of 1962.

As the years progressed and the breeders tried to breed healthy, sighted collies, the breeders finally reached a point where the perspective collie parents were all checked for PRA. Once PRA was not found or identified, their breeding programs started to eliminate this genetic defect. Good for them, because it showed that they really cared for the breed.

Other breeds, like Scottish Terriers, have developed another genetic defect, Sudden Acute Retinal Degeneration Syndrome (SARDS). Usually by the time the pet owner realizes his or her pet is having visual problems, the damage has been done.

Routinely, Plechner's Syndrome is tested for and controlled before this autoimmune disease will cause permanent retinal damage. The problem needs to be recognized as soon as possible. If your pet seems to have a slight vision problem at night and no cataract lenses or lens capsule opacities, SARDS must be considered. A visit to your veterinarian or veterinary ophthalmologist will be important.

If you bought a blue-eyed Persian cat, there is a good chance the cat was deaf. Again, just one more genetic breeding defect caused by man.

A number of years ago, Doberman Pinschers developed a genetic disorder causing a lack of blood clotting, which led to the bleeding disorder called Von Willebrand's Disease.

Other breeds, along with Doberman Pinschers, began developing enlarged hearts, called cardiomegaly. I was given the opportunity to help the breeder of a line of Dobermans to get rid of this problem in the breeding program. A certain amino acid had been used to try to prevent this problem, called taurine. It might have been of some help, but it did not stop the hearts from enlarging to the point of heart failure. Taurine does help cats to not develop a cardiomyopathy that can develop without this nutrient. I am sure we see this disease occurring due to genetic effects in breeding programs.

I was the first person to create a rabbit and rice formulation for Nature's Recipe Pet Foods with eight hundred milligrams of taurine in the nutritional formulation. Many other pet food manufacturers had never done this before and did not realize that when chicken heart was included in the byproducts that they put in their pet food, that it probably contains a higher concentration of taurine than any other food supplement beside adding taurine itself. This is the main reason a taurine addition is often prescribed for dogs with enlarged hearts or for families of dogs where there is a fear of future heart enlargement.

English bulldogs have genetically induced problems with cleft lips and palates and with undescended testicles. At one time, in England, the undescended testicle problem became so widespread that the dog show judges allowed a bulldog to be shown with only one testicle. Just one more story of the quest for man to gain ribbons and cups at the expense of his dogs' health!

Those people who breed for function unfortunately got into the same situation; however, it developed more slowly. The dogs were bred for function like for sight, scent, agility, and stamina. There were certain strains of a breed that demonstrated that they had it all. Obviously, people would breed the "best of the best," but unfortunately, when the gene pool became too close, genetic defects occurred.

It was often thought that line breeding was the only way to create function with structure. Wrong! When grandfather or grandmother were bred to the granddaughter or grandson or niece and nephew, major genetic defects accompanied. If you realize the inherent genetic defects that would come into your family if you did this, then why would you use this sort of defective breeding program with your pets?

Many times it has been learned that genetic out-crossing may help. What is not realized is that if you try to use a dog from another country, usually they have carried out the same line breeding techniques that were done here in the United States.

A veterinarian should be able to easily predict genetic defects that might affect any breed a client might be considering to bring into his or her family. There are many breed-specific and non-breed-specific genetic conditions that may accompany a specific breed.

I would encourage my client and his family to go to an all-breed dog show and provide me with a list of all the breeds they might be considering. This then allows me to speak to them about specific genetic defects that might accompany their choices of a breed to bring into their family. Then I can indicate to them what may lie ahead for the family financially to keep this breed healthy from a medical standpoint.

There is nothing as sad for me, as a veterinarian, as to have a small child standing in front of me, holding a pet dying from a genetic defect, saying, "Please help me," when I know I can't!

I have been a conservationist for over five decades. I created and supported a wildlife rehabilitation center in the Santa Monica Mountains of Southern California called Stonewood Meadows, and I was also the volunteer research immunologist for the Big Horn Sheep Society of California. With the help of the Big Horn Sheep Society of California, we were able to translocate eleven ewes and lambs and two beautiful rams to Independence, California.

This work gave me the opportunity to take blood samples from the sheep to make sure that the transplants did not have any of the markers for Plechner's Syndrome. This gave us confidence through this blood test that they carried complementary genetics, before we put this breeding stock back into the environment. The history of bighorn sheep shows us how man's progress with railways, highways, and fences definitely stopped the chances for new gene pools to be created—the bands of wild sheep could no longer roam due to these obstacles. Therefore, a non-roaming dominant ram or his offspring son pretty much "ruled the roost." Unfortunately, this caused the gene pool to become too close. I did the blood test I developed for Plechner's Syndrome on all of the bighorn sheep that were to be trans located to Independence California. The testing was done to determine if their genetics had become too close and their survival could be limited due to this disorder. The tests indicated that this was not the case and the translocation went to completion.

In Africa, with free-ranging wildlife, it has become of major importance to protect the predators, (hyenas, jackals, wild dogs, etc.) because by having the predators available to chase the herds around, there will be no dominant males, and the gene pool will be diversified enough to keep the herds healthy.

This will hopefully help you to understand the problems of today and the future that we face with all animals, whether they are domestic or wildlife.

Man has completely altered our animals' environment and, after we have decimated certain species and completely altered their environment, we try to reintroduce back into that environment nonnative species for our own enjoyment and as a possible making of amends for having forced our other native species into a crisis state.

Any time man decides to attempt to benefit the environment via the work of environmental activists and agencies, they need to carefully consider the results that they may achieve before starting their work. The reintroduction of a native or nonnative species into an altered environment usually will have adverse consequences.

To not allow proper management of a wilderness area is criminal. The forests need proper management, as do our wildlife. Just because it is a tree or a plant, don't let man kill its future! The trees in the forest also develop diseases that can wipe out miles and miles of forest. If mature trees cannot be selectively harvested, seedlings and young trees will not be allowed enough sunlight to grow properly.

The undergrowth plus noxious weeds need management to stop the damage that these noxious weeds do to seedlings, small trees, and usable habitat for our wildlife.

Most environmentalists assume that if a wilderness area is left alone, it will better itself and survive; therefore, there is no reason to manage the trees and the wildlife that used to call their wilderness area home. **Wrong!**

It is a shame that people with so little knowledge and experience have made such a huge impact on our failing environment.

If people are so knowledgeable and self-serving that they need to enter a species of nonnative animals back into this altered environment, they need to try to determine by working with real wildlife experts how many pairs of this species should be released. It is apparent to me that frequently the pairs that are released back into an altered environment should be spayed or neutered before being released. Doing this will determine their impact on the environment without increasing the size of the release. Once this is has been determined by the experts, a certain number of fertile pairs might be released.

Do the wolf releases in Idaho, Wyoming, and Colorado ring a bell?

I love wolves. As a matter of fact, I used to volunteer to help the wolf colony in San Jacinto, California, many years ago. I also love deer, elk, and moose.

Unfortunately, with the wolf releases in the three different states, once they were reintroduced, they created enough offspring that they overwhelmed and killed many of the native wildlife and domestic species. In many areas, the resident wildlife being killed has caused the rest of the wildlife to look for new areas in order to survive.

My hope is that our native wildlife species can survive and, hopefully, so can the wolves.

Unfortunately, the damage has been done, and now the wolves can again be legally hunted. This entire scenario is sad for both the wildlife and the wolves. The wolves never ask to be transplanted and released. This is just another example of man's way of helping Mother Nature.

Fifty Years of Healing

I am thankful for all of the work of the conservation groups around the world that are trying to reverse the bad effects that man has caused to our environment. Believe me when I tell you that the conservation efforts for wildlife and the work for the ethical breeding of pets will succeed as we try to guarantee a better world for animals, ourselves, and our children for many generations to come.

The Genetic Ice Age

The "Genetic Ice Age" is how I think about the gradual breakdown of us, our animals, and our earth.

As this gradual breakdown is occurring, a concentration of the predisposing factors leading to poor health are being created. Not only are we seeing entire families of people developing allergies, autoimmunity and cancer, but we are seeing an even faster progression of disease in our animals due to indiscriminant breeding and breeding without functional purpose.

The lack of concern for our earth has further allowed for environmental breakdown, contamination of our soils and waters, and the development of an unstable atmosphere. We are potentially destroying our own lifeline.

With this present-day, slowly progressing destruction, a potentially dangerous cortisol deficiency is being created, which allows the immune system to not protect people and animals as designed, but rather allows for the loss of recognition of the body's own tissue by these cells, resulting in allergies, autoimmunity, cancer, and other ill effects. This disorder is what others have named Plechner's Syndrome.

The identification and control of this syndrome may slow down the slowly progressing ice age that is upon us.

Review and Summary

The following are the facts that I hope you have learned by reading this text.

Cortisol is a natural hormone secretion, in both you and your pet, produced by the middle layer of the adrenal cortex. This may turn out to be the most vital hormone produced in the body. When deficient or defective, it may lead to allergies, autoimmunity, and cancer.

Any amount of cortisol measured in twenty-four hours does not indicate that the cortisol is active or bound. Twenty-four-hour urine tests and salivary tests are performed to demonstrate the amount of free cortisol, as with other free hormones. These tests measure free cortisol; however, without relating its level to antibody production, you cannot tell if the free cortisol or any other free hormone can be used by the body.

When cortisol is deficient, defective, or bound, storage thyroid, T4, is not transferred into active thyroid, T3. This effective cortisol imbalance can be one reason why a pet or pet owner can become hypothyroid.

When long-term medical treatment for a cortisol imbalance is called for medically, normally there is no concern about a bound thyroid or a lack of thyroid hormone transference from storage thyroid to active thyroid. As the daily physiological cortisol replacement dose is given, due to the dysfunctional thyroid that is not working, the metabolism of the liver is decreased, causing a small amount of replacement cortisol to remain in a twenty-four-hour period. After one to two weeks, what was once a physiological dose of replacement cortisol has now turned into a harmful, long-term pharmacological dosage level.

I personally believe that the bad reputation that long-term cortisol replacement has gained is due to the fact that health care professionals do not realize that with long-term cortisol therapy, they must include a thyroid hormone to stop the buildup of the cortisol to physiologically harmful levels.

There are species variations that need to be recognized. During long-term cortisol therapy, dogs need a twice-daily T4 replacement. Cats usually do not need a T4 replacement unless they have feline infectious peritonitis (FIP). Horses do not routinely need a cortisol replacement and usually take only a T4 replacement, which allows for an increased metabolism of the hormones produced by the middle layer of the adrenal cortex that increases production of their own natural cortisol. People, at times, require both a T3 and T4 hormone replacement.

Something for you to think about for yourself: if you have a cortisol imbalance, which causes a reduced transference from T4 to T3, and you are told to take a T4 replacement for your hypothyroidism, can you understand why you still may be hypothyroid?

Total estrogen levels at the proper level are vital to having good health for you and your pet. Universally, you will find good health is created by a normal ratio between active cortisol and total estrogen.

Total estrogen includes the following:

- Estrogen from the ovaries

- Estrogen from the inner layer adrenal cortex in both males and females

- Estrogens from plants, referred to as phytoestrogens

- Estrogens from plastics, referred to as xenoestrogens

- Pesticides and chemicals that act as estrogens

- Estrogens from medications, supplements, groundwater, and municipal water sources

Excess adrenal estrogen comes from a lack of active cortisol or from other sources containing estrogen.

Excess estrogen binds active thyroid hormone. This is just another way both you and your pet can have normal levels of T3 and T4, and still both be hypothyroid.

When a hypothyroid condition is present, for whatever reason, the metabolism of the liver is reduced, as is the excretion rate of the kidneys. In this instance, the liver cannot process cholesterol effectively; a cholesterol excess can occur even with a cholesterol-modified diet.

Excess estrogen also deregulates both the T and B lymphocytes in the immune system. The T cell protects you and your pet against viruses and molds and fungi. The B cell protects you and your pet against bacteria and not only produces antibody to foreign invaders but also produces protective antibodies to vaccines.

When both the T lymphocyte and B lymphocyte are deregulated, they not only lose their ability to protect you, but they lose their recognition of self tissue and will attack the body, causing autoimmunity and cancer. When this deregulation occurs, destruction may occur to the red blood cells, white blood cells, platelets, nerve and muscle tissue, and almost any tissue in the body.

To add further problems for you and your pet, once the deregulation of the B lymphocyte has occurred, all antibody production is decreased. When this occurs, production of the mucous membrane antibody (IgA) drops below a certain level and malabsorption occurs. When this happens, almost all oral medications, supplements, vitamins, and foods will not get into the bloodstream. Oral correction of this imbalance may become impossible without the use of intramuscular injections to bypass the malabsorptive intestines.

A prime example of this happening is when you or your pet is in the hospital on intravenous or intramuscular injections of medication, but when you are sent home with the same oral medications, the original disease returns. What happened? No one checked the IgA levels to see if oral absorption was possible in the present status of the patient. Don't you think it might be important to check a patient's IgA with a routine blood test to make sure the oral medications sent home can be assimilated by the patient? I refer to this protective mechanism, for this hormonal imbalance, as the vicious cycle.

Elevated estrogen levels also cause inflammation of the lining cells of arteries, referred to as endothelial cells. This elevation can lead to many disorders throughout the body, often causing excess levels of liver and muscle enzymes. Many professional health care institutions still teach that elevations of liver enzymes come from the use of a cortisol replacement. The term that they use to describe this condition is steroid hepatopathy.

Prednisone is a commonly used steroid by most of the medical professions. Prednisone must go through the liver to be converted to prednisolone. If there happens to be a liver disorder, the conversion is incomplete or ineffective, and the prednisone is not as effective pharmacologically, as not enough prednisolone as is required can be produced.

With the concern that the medical profession has with steroid hepatopathy, why isn't prednisolone used instead of prednisone to bypass the liver?

There is a large amount of clinical evidence that points to the fact that many of the patients that have increased elevations in liver and muscle enzymes have excess estrogen, causing inflammation of the lining cells of the arteries that carry blood to these organs. When an elevated state of estrogen is present, it has to make you wonder if this inflammation of the endothelial cells of the arteries leads to arteriosclerosis and atherosclerosis.

In women who have elevated adrenal estrogen, when their ovaries are also producing estrogen, the increased level of total estrogen will cause an inflammation of their cerebral arteries; due to this, many times they will experience not only migraine headaches but also epileptic seizures.

Plechner's Syndrome can be identified in parents, whether dogs, cats, or humans. In the case of dogs and cats, if the parents have a slight defect in the same area, that defect will be concentrated in the offspring, which may cause major health problems for the puppies or kittens during their lifetimes.

In order to stop these genetic defects in dog and cat parents, do the Plechner's Syndrome test, and find a different mate, even one that can be off, but just not off in the same area. This will usually allow the genetic defects to be bred out.

Puppies or kittens can be tested at eight to twelve weeks of age just for the four hormones to determine if anything needs to be funded to avoid future diseases. This can also be done with any puppy or kitten that may be new to your household.

As far as humans are concerned, it would be important to do this test before having a child so that you might head off some genetic defects that have come from the parents to their offspring.

It might give your pediatrician an idea as to what disorders to look for. Also, once the maternal hormones are out of the infant's system, the infant should have his or her endocrine levels checked to see if anything needs to be corrected immediately before a medical effect occurs later in the child's infancy.

The serum sample must be spun down and refrigerated immediately after it is taken from the patient. The sample needs to be kept refrigerated from the time the sample is taken, during shipping to the laboratory, and at the time the sample is being processed.

One day, health care professionals will provide the standard of including a temperature strip to accompany all blood samples. If the temperature of the sample exceeds a certain temperature level, then processing the sample is not only worthless to the health care professional and patient, but it is a waste of money. It is apparent if the sample became overheated because all of the hormone levels will be high, as well as the various antibodies.

If testing the serum for IgA, IgM, IgG levels, and they vary—one immunoglobulin is deficient, one is normal, and one is high—the laboratory has very likely processed the serum incorrectly. This is usually due to lab error. If all the antibodies are high, and the disorder does not involve a specialized immune disease, then the serum sample was definitely overheated somewhere in its travel.

Last, but not least, for you and your pet to maintain optimum endocrine-immune health, you need to keep a normal balance between active cortisol and total estrogen.

The Doan Family Speaks Out

(Clients of Dr. Alfred Plechner, DVM)

As we buried our second Shih Tzu within two months' time, we realized that something must be terribly wrong. The oldest dog of nearly thirteen years, named Mowgli, had suffered most of his life with chronic, painful ear infections, which were now beyond conventional means of medical help. The younger dog of nearly twelve years, named Milo, had always suffered from aggressive behavior; we were told by our vet, when he was just a little puppy, to either have his teeth ground down to the gumline or to euthanize him. We were horrified at the thought of putting a little puppy down, so we had his teeth ground down to his gumline, which turned his eyes white and nearly blinded him from the trauma. This only prevented puncture wounds and never lessened his aggression. As time went on, Milo became too aggressive and seemingly overnight was covered in planter warts. At that point, all we could think about was the safety and well-being of our children, and we felt that we had no other option than to euthanize him as well. Suddenly, our affectionately known "Shih Tzu boys" were gone.

What remained behind were images in our minds as to what seemed like so much more life still left in them, despite their illnesses, despite their ages. Since, as a family of five, we had all been suffering from the negative effects of hypothyroidism and adrenal insufficiency, it seemed logical to us to approach our vets with the idea that perhaps our dogs were suffering from the same issues. We addressed these same issues with our two vets, prior to their deaths, and we were told that it was just old age that they were suffering from. Not at all satisfied with the answer, we began to research on our own.

In the meantime, we had added to our family two Old English Sheepdog puppies, named Montana and Melodei, who are siblings. Immediately, we noticed the same aggressive behavior as we had seen previously in Milo while they played together. We also couldn't understand why they slept so much. We were surprised to see the tartar buildup on both of their upper and lower teeth, and their cracked paw pads that looked extremely painful to walk on. Just like Mowgli, Melodei had developed an ear infection that wouldn't go away, despite treatment, and both puppies' ears became infested with ear mites despite meticulous grooming. We were most concerned with Montana, who was beginning to have seizures and who was becoming unpredictably aggressive as he experienced them.

With the Lord's help, we came across www.drplechner.com. In an email, we explained everything that had happened to our Shih Tzu boys and what was currently going on with our new puppies. Dr. Alfred Plechner, DVM, quickly responded and informed us that it was his opinion that, despite the ages of our Shih Tzu boys, they could have been spared euthanasia. We were speechless! He also suggested that our new puppies were showing signs of an endocrine-immune imbalance, and he further suggested that it had taken the lives of our late Shih Tzu boys. He then suggested that we try his endocrine-immune imbalance protocol (a method based upon his forty-plus years of veterinarian experience and research) to fix their imbalances in cooperation with our current veterinarian. We took a leap of faith and, in cooperation with our current veterinarian, got their blood work done (known as the endocrine-immune panel (EI-1 panel), and were astonished at what we found out when the puppies' lab results came back.

The blood work measured the puppies' total estrogen levels (estriol, estradiol and estrone), T4 and T3 (functions of the thyroid), cortisol (a chemical produced in the outer layer of the adrenal gland that is used for energy and a strong immune system), and their IgA, IgG, and IgM (immunity) levels. Even though they had both been neutered and spayed a month and a half prior to their blood draws, *both* dogs showed very high total estrogen levels—including Montana, the male puppy! And their IgA, IgG, and IgM levels were very low. The diagnosis was so simple! The total estrogen was binding up any thyroid and adrenal functions and thereby causing their immunities to drop, leaving them unbalanced in their endocrine-immune systems. This had revealed itself in their outward symptoms of aggression, sleepiness, excessive tartar, cracked paw pads, and ear infections, along with a susceptibility toward ear mite infestations and seizures. So our next question was, "Why were their bodies making so much total estrogen in the first place?"

Dr. Alfred Plechner explained that in his forty-plus years of veterinarian experience he had seen this situation occur countless times worldwide. He reasoned from his extensive experience and research that the puppies' adrenal glands were either injured (from physical injuries or exposure to toxins) or that there was a genetic defect that enabled their adrenal glands to produce excessive amounts of total estrogen instead of the needed cortisol for energy and a strong immune system. He then suggested that we try his endocrine-immune imbalance protocol to break up and reduce their high levels of total estrogen. Once again, in cooperation with our current veterinarian, we immediately began treatment to break up their high levels of total estrogen. We are so glad that we did! Our puppies' aggression dropped dramatically, and they became playful and affectionate, which was a tremendous relief with children in our home. Their sleepiness turned to only occasional naps when needed. Their excessive tartar was fascinating to see when it turned from its very hard, bright yellow state to a sticky, white paste that was easily removed to expose beautiful, shiny white teeth underneath. Melodei's ear infection quickly recovered—what a relief to see her ear turn from being swollen, inflamed, and red in color to a normal-sized ear that was now a beautiful pink color. Their ear mite infestations quickly went away. Their paw pads become smoother. Montana's seizures suddenly stopped. We were overjoyed with the results!

Seeing the positive lab results combined with the positive physical results of our puppies, we began to wonder if such a protocol would work for people. After years of suffering from misdiagnosis, we approached our current physician concerning Dr. Alfred Plechner's human endocrine-immune imbalance protocol. Our current physician agreed to give it a try since all our previous efforts with many other physicians and specialists had given either little or no positive results. We took yet another leap of faith, in cooperation with our current physician, and had our (the parents) blood work done. We were tested for the human endocrine-immune panel and were once again astonished at what we found out when our lab results came back. *Both* of us had very high levels of total estrogen and low levels of IgA, IgM, IgG. Once again, it explained why our thyroid and adrenal replacement therapy wasn't working—*the total estrogen was binding everything that we tried to take to get well!* Once again, we asked the question as to where all this total estrogen was coming from.

Dr. Alfred Plechner explained once again that in his forty-plus years of veterinarian experience he had seen this situation occur countless times worldwide, and not just with animals but also with people. He reasoned from his extensive experience and research that our adrenal glands were either injured from physical injuries or exposure to toxins, or that there was a genetic defect that enabled our adrenal glands to produce excessive amounts of total estrogen instead of the needed cortisol for energy and a strong immune system. Once that happens, the whole endocrine-immune imbalance begins and the patient begins to suffer the ill effects. Some possible human ill effects, as seen in animals, may be related to adrenal fatigue/insufficiency, allergies, autoimmune disease, cancer, chronic ear, nasal, and respiratory infections, epilepsy, estrogen dominance, fibromyalgia, heart disease, hyper/hypothyroidism, infertility, irritable bowel syndrome, multiple miscarriages, and possible adverse vaccine reactions. Please see Research Articles on www.drplechner.com for more information on these and other possible human ill effects.

Basic suggestions on how to get our bodies' endocrine-immune imbalances back into balance are listed in Dr. Alfred Plechner's "Compendium of Articles: Endocrine-Immune Mechanisms in Animals and Human Health Implications" found on www.drplechner.com. Once again, in cooperation with our current physician, we immediately began treatment to break up our high levels of total estrogen. Slowly, since a person's overall system is not as fast in recovery as an animal's, we have started feel some relief from our ill effects of an unbalanced endocrine-immune system. My husband has felt a dramatic relief from the sharp pains that he had suffered from for several months in his left leg. As for me, after having suffered for over twenty years from severe allergy symptoms from fall allergies—specifically to goldenrods—I did not experience *any* allergy symptoms this year after having started the treatment, despite the overabundance of goldenrods in our area. We also started to experience a slow increase in our energy levels as well. And through our lab results, our total estrogen levels have dropped, and our IgA, IgG, IgM levels have started to come up. Recently, our three children also took the human endocrine-immune panel blood test and are in the very early stages of treatment since endocrine-immune imbalances may also occur in children.

Having tried everything else for our pets, as well as for our family, and having quickly run out of options, we are truly grateful that such an endocrine-immune imbalance protocol exists. It is improving our entire family's health, right down to our pets. We are convinced that the endocrine-immune imbalance protocol, researched and suggested by Dr. Alfred Plechner, DVM, actually works. We can say such a thing because we have seen firsthand the positive lab results, combined with the positive physical results, first in our puppies and then in ourselves. We wholeheartedly recommend Dr. Alfred Plechner's, endocrine-immune imbalance protocol for your pets and for you! We also recommend him because, to us, he's the doctor that never stops caring.

Mr. & Mrs. Hayden and Sheila Doan Madeleine, Mareinne, and Mareille Doan Puppy kids, Montana and Melodei, of Grand Blanc, Michigan

[Editor: Subsequent to this documentation, the Doan family learned, through the testing of their well water at Dr. Plechner's suggestion, that it was tainted with arsenic. There is little doubt that this was the environmental toxin that Dr. Plechner suspected was interfering with the normal function of all of their endocrine systems. With the removal of this toxin from their diets, they have all returned to normal health as of last contact.]

Index

Lightning Source UK Ltd.
Milton Keynes UK
UKOW051828281012

201323UK00015B/66/P